Unlimited Energy Now

By Catherine Carrigan

Table of Contents

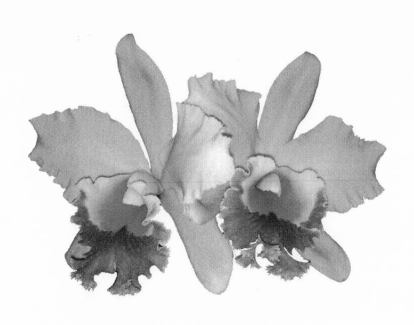

Introduction

Forward
You Can Get Better

"It always seems impossible until it's done." Nelson Mandela

Sometimes we wonder if we are ever going to get better, does the possibility even exist.

We also believe "If I just work harder and harder maybe I will have that time to make for my healing."

With adrenal exhaustion becoming the norm in society, it behoves you to listen to what this book is telling you.

The uniqueness of this book is that it puts into everyday perspective and language the "how to" of healing.

Your unique self has to read, listen to the advice and then take action, even if it is the smallest step and now you will be moving in the healing direction!

Catherine Carrigan has looked at all the different ways to clear the problem—Physical, Energetic, Mental, Emotional and Spiritual.

After you have identified for yourself the area you need the most, you no longer have to wonder how...just follow the directions.

The "how" can no longer be an excuse you use. Your soul energy will recognize this information as truth.

Your soul energy has been trying to nudge you in the right direction and now you have it in your hands.

Be very grateful for the nudge and continue to listen and grow and heal.

As a self empowerment coach myself, I see how *Unlimited Energy Now* will give you the results you are looking for and I would be surprised if you didn't share it with all you love!

Sue Maes, Self Empowerment Coach, Medical Intuitive

Chapter 1

The Gift of Unlimited Energy Now

"If you want to find the secrets of the universe, think in terms of energy, frequency and vibration." Nikola Tesla

What would you do if you had access to unlimited energy? My intention with this book is to empower you to experience unlimited energy *now.*

When you are blessed with unlimited energy:
You enjoy everything you do.
What you once thought of as depression becomes a distant memory.
Work that once felt tremendously challenging gets accomplished easily.
You radiate vitality.
You are an excellent partner, parent, daughter, son, sister, brother and friend.

You naturally bless others with your presence, as chi has its own intelligence and knows where it needs to go.
You love your life and give thanks for all you receive.

In my practice, the number one complaint I hear from virtually all of my new clients is fatigue.

I have spent years empowering clients to rebuild themselves after adrenal burnout, lifelong depression, serious illness, chronic fatigue and all manner of pain that was once thought incurable.

Unwinding these patterns as a medical intuitive healer, I have found that certain truths must be faced on each level of our existence:

1. You can operate your body at a higher level.
2. You can master your own energy system.
3. You can process your emotions and stop the pattern of being drained by the past.
4. You can tell yourself better stories from the vantage point of an empowered, authentic human.
5. Your soul can connect even more deeply to experience constant, unwavering unconditional support from all that is.

As we work through all these levels - the physical, energetic, emotional, mental and spiritual - my clients not only restore their prana but also rediscover who they really truly are.

Chapter 2
My Personal Recovery from Exhaustion

"Be still and know that I am God." Psalm 46:10

I remember distinctly the day I received the lab results.

Months before then, I had prepaid for a two-week bike tour of Ireland and was due to leave within the next two weeks. The medical doctor who explained the report to me explained that I was in stage 3 of stage 3 of adrenal stress, the very final stage of total exhaustion.

The next stage after that would be death.

Yes, I had been teaching yoga and qi gong, taking vitamins, eating healthy, and engaging in all manner of positive health processes.

I hadn't been doing anything wrong, I just wasn't getting anywhere.

All the good work I had been doing felt like it was being poured into a bottomless black hole.

I looked fluffy and mildly overweight in sort of a pathetic middle-aged way.

No matter how little I ate, I was not able to regain my usual trim, athletic figure.

My memory was fuzzy but I had been muddling through my work with my usual focus, determined not to give up no matter what.

The doctor advised me not to ride my bicycle at all on the upcoming trip.

Not only did I not ride my bike, the most I did the entire trip was take one 30-minute walk.

Even that felt like way too much, and I spent most of the trip trying to recover from the plane ride overseas, which wiped me out so badly I spent the first 24 hours in Ireland just sleeping.

When I returned from my trip, I made the decision to turn the corner.

The trip had felt like one big uncomfortable blur - not exactly a true vacation.

It was like walking to the edge of a cliff and gazing over to oblivion.

I had been given a blessing.

Someone had waved a large, invisible but unmistakable stop sign in my face.

I stopped, paused and listened.

Since that day I have done whatever it takes to rebuild my personal energy, and, in the process, come to value this thing that people call variously life energy, prana, chi, life force, vitality.

Although our life energy is indeed invisible, we know when we have it and are also painfully aware when we don't have it.

I learned how to experience unlimited energy now.

As I have been blessed, I share this blessing with you, my dear reader.

This is my book about how you can also experience unlimited energy right now in a healthy, easy way.

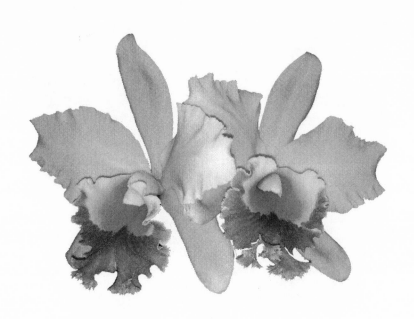

Book One

The Ultimate Athlete Hidden Inside of You: The Physical Body

Chapter 1

Your Adrenal Glands, Stage 1 Alarm Phase

"I have chosen to be happy because it is good for my health." Voltaire

Inside your body, you have two adrenal glands. They sit on top of your each kidney and secrete your stress hormones, cortisol and adrenalin.

When your adrenal glands begin to be challenged, your energy shifts.

Stage 1 of adrenal stress is the beginning of the problem.

Stage 1 is characterized by:

1. Stress stimulation
2. Activation of your sympathetic nervous system
3. Your body releases adrenalin and cortisol

4. You experience a stress response, which may be characterized by the following symptoms:

*Increased heart rate
*Constriction of blood vessels of your skin and gastrointestinal tract
*Conversion of glycogen to glucose
*Contraction of your spleen
*Sweating
*Dilation of your bronchial tubes
*Decrease in your digestive processes
*Decreased urine production
*Anxiety
*Depression
*Agitation/irritability
*Restless sleep
*Increased cholesterol
*Increased triglycerides
*Impaired memory/learning

Techniques that work to turn around stage 1 include:

1. Recognize that you are being challenged and take the steps necessary to take your life at an easier pace.
2. Eat five small meals every day to keep your blood sugar balanced.
3. Meditate.
4. Exercise daily.
5. Go to bed, lights out, no later than 10:30 p.m.

6. Taking the steps necessary to sleep soundly through the night.
7. Daily stress management.

Chapter 2

Your Adrenal Glands, Stage 2 Adaptation Phase

"How you vibrate is what the universe echoes back to you in every moment." Panache Desai

Beginning in stage 2 of adrenal stress, you may notice that your metabolism seems to have changed. Your ability to metabolize carbohydrates and fat has altered. If you go to your medical doctor, he may mention that your thyroid has been acting up. You may retain water and feel more tired on an ongoing basis. Your ability to respond to day to day stresses seems to be diminished.

Other signs and symptoms of stage 2 of adrenal stress:

*Your metabolic rate seems to have slowed down
*You seem to have accepted the fact that your life is just plain stressful
*Weight gain

*Fatigue
*Cold intolerance
*Memory loss
*Poor concentration
*Depression
*Muscle weakness and stiffness
*Menstrual irregularities
*Digestive disorders

You will need to be more consistent for a longer period of time to heal stage 2 of adrenal stress. To have gotten to this point physiologically, you have been stressed for a longer period of time.

Strategies that help for stage 2 of adrenal stress include:

1. Daily stress reduction activities.
2. Meditation.
3. Bed and lights out no later than 10:30 p.m.
4. Five mini meals throughout the day to keep your blood sugar balanced.
5. Mental/emotional clearing work to identify the issues that have been driving you. This may include psychological therapy or kinesiology sessions to root out the key issues.
6. Develop hobbies that bring balance into your life.
7. Re-examine your work schedule. Remember, if you work too hard at your job you may be allowing someone else to steal your personal chi.

8. If you are an introvert, give yourself permission to take time alone to regenerate.
9. If you are an extrovert, make plans for ongoing group activities to regenerate.
10. Regular consistent exercise, up to but no more than 1 hour every day.
11. Take time off to rest.

Chapter 3

Stage 3 of Adrenal Stress, Exhaustion

"There is only one corner of the universe you can be certain of improving, and that's your own self." Aldous Huxley

By the time you have gotten to stage 3 of adrenal stress, you have ignored all the obvious stop signs.

I explain to my clients that getting to stage 3 is like driving down the road, seeing a stop light or stop sign, and saying to yourself, "I am so busy and important. That stop sign doesn't apply to me!"

At this point, you have ignored your body's own signals for so long that you may have developed degenerative diseases.

Signs and symptoms that you are in stage 3 of adrenal stress include:

*Inability to lose weight no matter how little you eat or how much you exercise
*Chronic fatigue
*Depression or anxiety not alleviated by antidepressants or talk therapy
*Severe body aches and pains
*Reproductive failure
*Immune suppression
*Poor ability to recover from exercise, injuries and illnesses
*Digestive disorders
*Hormonal depletion
*Weight gain around your midsection
*Inability to cope
*Chronic pain
*Reduced libido
*Severe allergies or asthma
*Fatigue not alleviated by normal sleep or rest

Strategies that help to get you out of stage 3 of adrenal stress include:

1. Daily mental/emotional stress reduction.
2. Naps.
3. Bed by 10:30 p.m.

4. Even though you are tired at this point, your brain chemistry may be so depleted that you may need supplements or medication to help you sleep.
5. Amino acids and/or protein supplements.
6. Grizzly. This is probably the most powerful technique, as you can take all the drugs and supplements you want but if you don't rest you can't actually improve. Ask your kinesiologist to muscle test to find out how many days of complete rest you will need to recover. Generally with people in stage 3 of adrenal stress, this may be as many as 20 to 40 days of complete rest.
7. In grizzly, the technique is simple. Spend as much time lying down as possible. If you fall asleep, great, as by this point you are also sleep deprived. You may read funny or spiritually uplifting books but no work material. You may bead, knit, crochet or needlepoint. You can do craft work. You can meditate, take a hot bath or watch funny or uplifting movies but not TV (which bombards you with commercials and violence).
8. Because stage 3 is usually accompanied by a feeling of spiritual depletion, I recommend finding a spiritual support group, church, mosque, synagogue, meditation group or some other spiritual community.
9. Begin forgiveness work, as lack of forgiveness acts like a heavy stone on your heart and blocks your prana like nothing else.
10. Psychological processing to release the emotions that have weighed you down.

11. Restrict your exercise to energy-building methods such as restorative yoga, tai chi, qi gong and/or walking until your vitality significantly improves.

Chapter 4
Alignment

"Spiritual energy flows in and produces effects in the phenomenal world." Williams James

As a yoga teacher for the past 18 years, one of the blessings I have received - both for myself and for my students - is what happens when you bring the body into structural alignment.

Here's a simple way to understand it:

Your physical body is the densest part of you.

There are also these other layers - your energy body, your emotions, your mind and your soul.

You can bring all these layers into balance by practicing alignment in the way you sit, stand and sleep.

Good posture is simply defined as the place in which you are most bio biomechanically efficient.

When you sit, stand and sleep with great posture, you can experience unlimited energy right *now.*

Let me put this in the converse. If you sit with your shoulders rounded forward, your head jutting into the future and your chest tightened, your lungs will collapse and it will be very hard for you to get a good breath.

Because your breath is the bridge between your mind and body, this shallow breathing will not only lead to low physical prana but also to a subpar emotional state.

Maybe you won't exactly feel depressed, but you won't feel like running around the block or leaping tall buildings either.

When you sit in this rounded, collapsed state, not only will you be low vibration emotionally, your mindset about yourself will also be diminished.

On the other hand, if you sit on your sit bones, chest spread, both sides of your body even with a slight arch in your lower back, your lungs can expand naturally.

Not only will you bring more oxygen into your brain, you will bring more necessary and essential nutrients to every cell in your body.

Most chronic diseases - such as cancer - happen in a low oxygen environment. When we take the time to sit properly, stand up properly and sleep with very good posture, we can bring healing oxygen to every cell.

How to sit for energy:

1. Find your sit bones.
2. Sit with a 30 to 35 degree arch in your lower back.
3. Put both feet flat on the floor.
4. Lift and expand your chest.
5. Pull your shoulder blades down towards your waist.

How to stand to feel great:

1. You can practice by putting a book between your feet. Hug the book with your feet to bring your feet into alignment. Your feet have to be pointing straight ahead in a relaxed position for your hips to be square and your knees to feel good. When you have your feet square, you can remove the book.
2. Remember: Your feet control your hips, your hips control your knees and your legs extend your spine. If you have any pain or discomfort anywhere, go higher up the chain. For example, if you have knee pain, put your hips into alignment by straightening your feet.
3. Pull your inner thighs back. Keep your knees soft.
4. From two inches below the belly button, lift the pit of your abdomen towards the crown of your head.
5. Lift and spread your chest.
6. Slide your shoulder blades towards the waist.
7. Make a fist with one hand. Place your fist between your chin and your chest to position your head properly. Remove your fist and keep your head on straight!

How to sleep for better energy:

1. If you have any back pain, lie on your side and put a pillow between your knees.
2. Support yourself with pillows until all your muscles can completely relax.

Chapter 5
Digestion, the Core of Gold

"Most people spend more time and energy going around problems than in trying to solve them." Henry Ford

One of the first things I focus on with clients who have depleted their life force is to restore digestion.

Why is your digestion so important?

*When your digestion is good, you bring animating force and nutrients to all your muscles, glands and organs.
*You can make your neurotransmitters, so that your brain can think straight and feel happy.
*You have a strong functioning immune system and balanced hormones.
On the other hand, if your digestion is in any way upset, you:

*May not be receiving the prana and nutrients your muscles, glands and organs require in order to work properly from food.

*May feel anxious and depressed because your brain chemistry is depleted.

*May pick up every cold and virus coming down the pike because your immune system is so depleted that you can't fight anything off.

*Your hormones may be in the tank.

*Your your sex drive may be nonexistent.

*You may be experiencing constant pain somewhere in the body, as about 70 percent of inflammation begins in your gut.

*You may feel ungrounded, incomplete or disempowered. Your digestion is the core of gold because when you fix your digestion, you can solve myriad other problems in your mind and body.

Many people are not aware that over 95 percent of your serotonin, your feel-happy brain chemical, is found in your gut. Your enteric nervous system (the nervous system in your gut) uses more than 30 neurotransmitters. http://www.scientificamerican.com/article/gut-second-brain/ If you want to check how your gut is doing, you will want to check four specific issues:

1. The functioning of your stomach
2. The degree of inflammation in your entire GI tract.
3. Your ability to secrete digestive enzymes

4. Whether or not you have bad bacteria, parasites, probiotic imbalances, incomplete digestion of food or other issues that are interfering.

Jeffrey Bland, Ph.D., developed what he calls the 4R program to heal your gut:

1. What needs to be removed?

*Toxins in food
*Food sensitivities or allergies
*GI irritants, such as coffee and alcohol
*Chronic low-grade infections

2. What needs to be replaced?

*Stomach acid
*Digestive enzymes

3. Does one need to re-inoculate with probiotics?

4. Does the intestinal lining need to be repaired?

http://www.drfranklipman.com/the-4r-program-to-promote-gastrointestinal-health/

Healing your digestive tract will restore your chi and even make it possible for you to get off antidepressant or anti anxiety medication. You may be surprised how your skin improves and how your endurance improves as a result of healing your stomach, intestines, pancreas and digestive system.

Chapter 6
Energy Exercise

"Failure is more frequently from want of energy than want of capital." Daniel Webster

We all know that exercise is good for us, but not all exercise is good for everybody.

If you are feeling tired on a regular and consistent basis, you may either not feel like exercising at all or find intense workouts making you feel worse.

That's because when your heart rate exceeds 100 beats per minute on a consistent basis, your body has to release the stress hormones cortisol and adrenalin to keep your heart rate above 100 beats per minute.

Kinds of exercise that may make you feel more depleted:

*Running
*Jogging

*Spinning classes
*Triathlons
*Boot camps
*Any exercise where your heart rate remains consistently elevated over 100 beats per minute.

On the other hand, activities such as weight training, where your heart rate is temporarily spiking upwards over 100 beats per minute and coming down again may be beneficial unless you are in stage 3 of adrenal stress.

Whatever stage of adrenal stress you are in, you can rebuild your chi by practicing energy exercise.

There are three primary forms of energy exercise:

*Yoga
*Tai Chi
*Qi gong

Why are these forms of exercise especially beneficial?

1. Yoga is designed to open and balance your chakras. When your chakras are open and balanced on a consistent basis, you will experience unlimited energy.
2. Tai chi works primarily on the acupuncture system. Both your chakras and your acupuncture meridians distribute energy through your body. You can visit an acupuncturist, which may be highly beneficial, or you can balance your own meridians by practicing tai chi.

3. Qi gong is a part of tai chi and also balances your acupuncture system. Qi gong exercises are generally less complex and easier to learn if you are feeling mentally overloaded.

4. Yoga, tai chi and qi gong lower your stress hormones. You will notice your energy goes up as your stress level goes down.

When you practice yoga, tai chi or qi gong, begin by giving yourself two numbers:

1. Your stress number, with 0 being no stress and 10 being high stress.

2. Your energy number, which 0 being none, totally exhausted, and 10 being high, clear vibration.

Check in with yourself midway through your practice and again at the end.

Even if you have not completely eliminated your stress and totally boosted your life force to a 10, most you will feel dramatically better.

Chapter 7
Great Clothes

"If you are depressed, get dressed." Adrienne Landau

One of the simplest and easiest ways to turn around the way you feel in an instant is to dress your best at all times.

Why does this make such a difference?

Your outside reflects what's happening on the inside.

At the same time, your inside also mirrors what's happening on the outside.

Dress like a bum, *feel* like a bum.

Dress like a bag lady, *feel* like a bag lady!

Whether you are a man or a woman, this advice may seem totally superficial until you take the time to discover what colors, materials and style of dress makes you feel the best.

1. If you are not good at knowing what clothes make you feel your best, ask for help. Call in a professional or a friend who really loves you.

2. Bring in large trash bags you can load up to donate to people who may need your old duds more than you do.

3. Go through your closets and throw out anything old that you haven't worn in over a year. If you haven't worn it in over a year, chances are it's old vibration that doesn't reflect where you are in your life right now.

4. Give away any attire that you have labeled as your "fat clothes." If you wear "fat clothes" every day, you are subconsciously agreeing with the message that you are not expressing your best self.

5. Give away any regalia that you wore at upsetting events, e.g., at a divorce closing, when you were fired, in an accident. Just like an actor changes his costume to assume a different role, this is an important step when you want to change your vibration.

6. Have your friend who is assisting you muscle test which outfits and accessories to keep (please see the appendix if you want to learn how to muscle test). You should stay strong with every garment you put on your body. Anything that makes you go weak is lowering your vibration every time you put it on, no matter how expensive, fashionable or memorable it may be.

7. Finally, put together at least four complete outfits - clothes, shoes, belts, scarves and total accessories -

that compliment your best features. You will know that when you wear them, you are expressing your highest version of yourself and feel most confident.

Chapter 8
Feng Shui

"A strong, successful man is not the victim of his environment. He creates favorable conditions." Orison Swett Marden

Just as dressing well on the outside can help you feel better on the inside, one very important way to regain your personal chi is by changing the Feng shui of your personal environment.

Environment is the most powerful factor.

Just as the most beautiful orchid can't bloom in a dark room without sunlight or water, so too you must place yourself in the most conducive environment for you to prosper.

When your house is full of dust and clutter that old energy acts as energetic stagnation and congestion.

You can't bring in anything new because the old energy is quite literally blocking the flow of your chi.

Often our home environments - like our clothes - reflect what is really happening on the inside.

If you want to actually see for yourself what's going on for you internally go to your bedroom - where you are probably spending at least 8 hours every night - and take a deep look.

Here are a few suggestions about how to improve your environment to maximize the flow of your personal energy:

1. If you live in an environment where the outside humidity is above 50 percent, I recommend you purchase a small portable home humidity monitor for about $10. Mold can grow in any environment where the humidity is 50 percent or above. Nothing will pull down your personal chi like living in literal rot. If you find that your home is full of mold, you can install a dehumidifier and take up mold remediation with the help of experts.
2. Give away any objects that you have not used in the past year.
3. Throw away everything that is broken that can't be fixed.
4. Give away any object that brings up a negative emotional charge. If you look at a photo of a person that you no longer resonate with, or glance at a vase

from your father you no longer speak with, your home is actually a hidden source of post traumatic stress disorder.

5. Clean your home weekly. Because dust is made up of 70 to 80 percent human skin, if you are not dusting, vacuuming and cleaning regularly, you are unconsciously stuck in the past.

6. Place living plants throughout your space.

7. Allow fresh air to circulate. Open the windows when the temperature permits.

8. Ask a friend to muscle test you in every room in your home (see the appendix if you want to learn how to muscle test). If you go weak, ask yourself what you need to add, balance or take away.

9. In Feng shui, they say if you want to change your life, change 27 things in your home environment. Paint, plant a garden, wash your windows or rearrange the furniture.

Everywhere you look, you want to be reminded in your home of how much you love others and are loved and cared about, how happy and fulfilling your life is and surround yourself with objects that make you feel comfortable, relaxed and supported.

Chapter 9

Grizzly, The Fastest Cheapest Way
to Recover Your Energy

"The secret of change is to focus all of your energy not on fighting the old, but on building the new." Socrates

When I am working with exhausted clients, I always use kinesiology to muscle test how many days of complete rest their body will need to restore their life force.

Although my repertoire includes nutritional supplements to support the adrenal glands, the fastest, cheapest way to get better if you are wiped out is to rest.

Here's how it works:

Step 1. Determine how many days of complete rest you will need to restore your energy. Even if you only rested one day each weekend, you could get 52 days of rest every year!

Step 2. Bring out your schedule. Even if you can only rest for half a day at a time, schedule out as many days of half days of complete rest until you have fulfilled your requirement. If you can take a week off, even better. It is not necessary to go on vacation. A stay cation at home often works even better so you can give yourself permission to do nothing - no sightseeing, no travel stress, no visits to unhappy relatives.

Step 3. Rest. You are allowed to:

*Read funny or uplifting books (no work material)
*Watch funny or uplifting movies (no TV with commercials)
*Nap
*Sleep
*Meditate
*Stretch
*Take a hot bath
*Hobbies that involves sitting, such as knitting, beading, needlework, quilting, needlepoint, woodworking, airplane making, drawing or painting
*Do absolutely nothing.

Chapter 10
Pain Blockages

"See where your own energy wants to go, not where you think it should go. Do something because it feels right, not because it makes sense. Follow the spiritual impulse."
Mary Hayes-Grieco

One of the things that you will notice is that when you suffer from pain you feel fatigued.

This is one of the reasons that getting rid of your pain is a necessary step to restore your chi.

Often, when we begin our healing journey, we turn to medications - either over the counter or prescription drugs.

Socrates said that people always choose the good. If you currently use medicines, either self-prescribed or from your doctor, do not blame yourself.

All medications have side effects. Look up the side effects of all your drugs at www.rxlist.com.

Even if you think you know, you may discover that the drugs you have been taking have been creating other side issues.

You can check the chi of any substance - whether it be a prescription drug, a vitamin, herb or food - by holding a pendulum over it.

Natural substances have higher life energy. If a substance is beneficial for you, your pendulum will spin clockwise.

A substance that is not in your highest best interests will spin backwards or not move at all, indicating that it depletes your life energy.

When we are in pain, it's important to find methods that actually work to relieve suffering without depleting our chi.

Pain antidotes that build your energy may include:

*Rest
*Ice
*Compression
*Elevation
*Massage
*Energy healing
*Epsom salt baths
*Juices made from fruits and vegetables to alkalize your body
*Fish oil to lower inflammation

*Water, as a common symptom of dehydration is pain anywhere in the body

*Turmeric, ginger, capsaicin, bromelain, feverfew, ginseng, boswellia, willow bark, kava kava or other natural substances. Ask your naturopath, nutritionist or kinesiologist what you can use instead of drugs.

Chapter 11
Sleep, A Balm for the Soul

"The universe is responding to your vibration, and your vibration is about the way that you feel." Abraham Hicks

In the back of your brain is a structure called your Reticular Activating System, your RAS.

Your Reticular Activating System or RAS is responsible for your sleep-wake cycle.

When we have experienced trauma, the RAS is hyper vigilant, always on the alert looking for anything that could potentially harm, injure, disrupt or unsettle us.

Because you have to calm this unconscious aspect of your brain in order to go to sleep, up to now, deep, restorative sleep may have eluded you.

Your physical body regenerates when you sleep from 10 p.m. to 2 a.m.

From 2 a.m. to 6 a.m., you rebuild your brain chemistry. You process your emotions and repair your mind.

Here are a few great steps you can take to sleep soundly:

1. Turn out your lights no later than 10:30 p.m., since every minute of sleep before midnight is worth 10 minutes of sleep after midnight.
2. Aim for a total of 10 hours of rest every day. For example, if you sleep for 8 hours, take a 30 minute nap, meditate for another 30 minutes, sit in a 30 minute hot bath and lie down and read a book for another 30 minutes.
3. If you find yourself worrying, interrupt the habit. Designate a time earlier in the day for worrying. At the appointed time, write down everything that concerns you. Then, when it is anything other than your designated worry time, stop the habit and redirect your focus.
4. Keep your body at least 6 to 8 feet away from electrical outlets that may interfere with your brain going into delta, the brain waves necessary for deep sleep.
5. If you tend to wake up in the middle of the night, you may be experiencing either high or low blood sugar. Eat a small, glycemically balanced snack right before bed. This should include some form of protein. A good choice is kefir mixed with strawberries, or turkey with an apple, as these combinations boost your serotonin. Serotonin is used by your brain to

make melatonin, the hormone that helps you sleep deeply.

6. Lower your stress level throughout the day. The stress hormone cortisol has a six-hour half life and interrupts sleep. If you become upset late in the day, your body may not have time to process enough cortisol so you can sleep deeply at night.

7. Pray or meditate before bed to set your mind at peace.

8. If you find you are grinding your teeth at night, you may have parasites. Ask your health practitioner to test your digestive system for parasites so you can stop the teeth grinding and relax.

9. Avoid alcohol before bed, as alcohol may interfere with your REM cycle.

10. Avoid caffeine after 4 p.m. It takes about 8 to 10 hours for your body to clear 75 percent of the caffeine you have consumed.

11. Avoid cigarettes and recreational drugs that disrupt your brain chemistry. Get professional help to heal your addictions.

12. Exercise during the day to release muscle tension. Avoid high intensity exercise that might raise your cortisol and adrenalin after 4 p.m. Practice yoga, tai chi or qi gong later in the day to lower your stress hormones.

13. Avoid TV, computers and the internet late at night. All of these stimulate your adrenal glands and may keep you awake.

14. Balance your blood sugar. Eat small meals 5 times throughout your waking hours including protein, fat, vegetables, and carbohydrates.

15. Heal your inflammation, which keeps cortisol levels high even at night. You can begin that process by cutting down on pro-inflammatory foods such as caffeine, alcohol, tobacco, sugar, gluten and fried foods.

16. Look up the side effects of all your medications. Make sure you are not taking anything that might interfere with your sleep.

17. Give thanks for all you have received throughout the day to lift your vibration as you go to sleep.

18. If your neck vertebrae are out of alignment, consider visiting a chiropractor. Often misalignments of your neck will keep you awake at night.

19. If you habitually have trouble falling asleep, have your amino acid levels tested. You may be deficient in the building blocks of your brain chemistry and unable to make the neurotransmitters necessary for deep sleep.

20. Keep a regular routine. Go to bed at the same time every night, even on the weekends, so that your body adapts to a healthy rhythm.

21. Keep televisions, cell phones, computers, and other electronic gadgets out of your bedroom. Keep your bedroom for two primary activities: sleep and sex.

22. Consult a Feng shui practitioner if your bedroom feels uncomfortable. Avoid mirrors in the bedroom.

Make sure your bed is not directly facing the door, which is known in Feng shui as "the death position."

23. Make sure you get at least 30 minutes of sunlight every day to stimulate your pineal gland to produce melatonin. Some people may need as much as 12 hours of sunlight daily. If you have a high need for sunlight and still aren't getting enough, consider testing your vitamin D levels and consult an alternative health care practitioner about other ways you can balance your body even if you don't get enough sunlight. You may want to consider a light box, which provides enough LUX to stimulate your natural melatonin production. This may be especially helpful if you tend to experience seasonal affective disorder, SAD, in the fall and winter.

24. Make sure your mattress is comfortable and supports your spine properly. If your bed is old and your back hurts, consider replacing it.

Chapter 12
Vibrant Food

"You are One with everything. When you are clear about this, your definition of self interest will change." Paramahansa Yogananda

You can experience unlimited energy right now by feeding your body a high life force diet.

Water

One of the quickest ways to boost your energy is to drink more water. The adult male human body is about 57 percent water. http://en.wikipedia.org/wiki/Composition_of_the_human_body

Symptoms of dehydration include:

- Fatigue
- High blood pressure

- Skin disorders
- Asthma and allergies
- High cholesterol
- Digestive disorders
- Bladder or kidney problems
- Constipation
- Joint pain and joint stiffness
- Weight gain
- Headaches
- Dizziness
- Your urine is more yellow than normal
- Dry mouth
- Tightness in your muscles
- Decrease in your strength
- Anxiety and depression, as all your neurotransmitters work in water
- Brain fog

Protein

Your body requires amino acids, the building blocks of protein, to make your neurotransmitters, muscles and connective tissue. Amino acid deficiencies are a common symptom of adrenal burnout and may be identified through lab tests.

Include some form of protein every time you eat in order to keep your blood sugar balanced.

Why is this so important? Carbohydrates alone raise your insulin, which regulates your blood sugar.

The hormone you have the most control is your insulin.

You can't heal your adrenal glands and overcome adrenal burnout if your insulin and blood sugar are out of balance.

Include organic, grass-fed sources of meat when possible to avoid antibiotics and hormones.

Healthy Carbohydrates, Fruits and Vegetables

Fruits and vegetables contain phytochemicals, biologically active compounds found in cellulose fiber that contain a wide array of healing properties.

Include these phytochemicals in your diet:

Alpha glucans, found in Shitake mushrooms: Boost your immune system and fight cancer.

Allicin, found in garlic: Kills viruses and bad bacteria.

Anthocyanins, found in blue and purple fruits and vegetables such as blueberries and purple sweet potatoes: One of nature's most powerful water-soluble antioxidants.

Beta carotene, found in highest concentrations in goji berries: Improves our eye and lung function and protects us from UV radiation.

Beta glucan, found in mushrooms: Lowers cholesterol.

Betain, found in beets: Lowers homocysteine levels and heals the heart.

Catechins, found in green and white tea: Natural blood thinners.

Charantin, found in bitter melon: Acts similar to insulin and keeps blood sugar balanced.

Chlorogenic acid, found in eggplant and green coffee beans: Improves fat metabolism.

Curcumin, found in turmeric: Keeps inflammation under control and lowers pain naturally.

D-Glucarate, found in grapefruit: Boosts your immune system and reverses cancer.

D-Mannose, found in cranberries: Clears urinary tract infections.

Ellagic acid, found in raspberries and strawberries: Causes cancer cells to die.

Ergothionine, found in Shitake and oyster mushrooms: Boosts energy by improving Phase II detoxification in your liver.

Ganoderic acid, found in Reishi mushrooms: Improves blood pressure, circulation and cholesterol.

Gingerol, found in ginger: Relieves pain and inflammation naturally.

Glucoraphanin, found in broccoli: Boosts your energy by supporting your Phase II detoxification in your liver.

Glutathione, found in highest concentration in asparagus: Boosts your energy by supporting Phase II detoxification in your liver.

Hydroxychalcone, found in cinnamon: Iimproves insulin handling.

Indole-3-Carbinol, found in cruciferous vegetables such as cauliflower: Improves estrogen metabolism and heals cancer.

Limonin, found in limes and the pith of all citrus fruits: A highly aggressive cancer fighter.

Lutein and Zeaxanthin, found in dark green and leafy vegetables such as spinach and kale: Supports the retina of your eyes.

Lycopene, found in watermelon and tomatoes: Supports the prostate and kidneys.

Natto, found in chard: The highest source of vitamin K1, helpful for anemia and blood thinning.

Orientin and vicenin, found in basil: Natural antioxidants.

Pectin, found in apples: Scrubs your arteries and improves bowel function.

Perillyl alcohol, found in mint: Stops tumor growth.

Phthalide, found in celery: Lowers blood pressure naturally.

Quercetin, found in capers: Heals skin issues.

Resveratrol, found in Muscadine grapes: Reduces inflammation.

Syringic acid, found in Swiss chard: Improves blood sugar handling.

I first learned about phytochemicals from George Mateljan, author of *The World's Healthiest Foods.* You can read more about his ongoing into the healing properties of natural foods at www.whfoods.com.

Most of what I learned about phytochemicals comes from Jeff Primack, author of *Conquering Any Disease.* Most people think of food simply in terms of calories or even vitamins and minerals. Jeff's approach to healing with food takes eating to a whole new level.

If you don't include enough carbohydrates in your diet, you may feel exhausted and depressed.

Dr. Diana Schwarzbein, M.D., an expert on metabolism, recommends you include at least 150 grams of carbohydrates every day.

If you have a damaged metabolism, you may need to cut back to 125 grams per day.

Include more carbohydrates if you are exercising.

To boost your unlimited energy, I recommend focusing on choosing the majority of your carbohydrates from fruits and vegtables because of their high antioxidant, high phytochemical properties.

Healthy Fats

Avocado: Rich in glutathione, which boosts Phase II detoxification in your liver and high in soluble fiber.

Butter and ghee: Rich in lecithin; essential for cholesterol metabolism as well as vitamins A, D, E and K2. Contains CLA, or Conjugated Linoleic Acid, which boosts your immune system.

Coconut oil: Best for high heat cooking. Boosts your immune system, anti-viral. Heals your thyroid.

Olive oil: Best used at room temperature. Eating olive oil with a meal reduces free radical production.

Walnuts: High in melatonin to help you sleep. Also high in Omega-3 fatty acids and L-arginine, which improve your circulation.

Chapter 13

Your Hormones Govern Your Behavior

"Please take responsibility for the energy you bring into this space." Dr. Jill Bolte Taylor

Ever try not to eat when you are very hungry?

Ever try to feel calm when you are in the midst of a panic attack?

Both of these events are accompanied by high levels of your stress hormone cortisol.

It takes six hours for half of the cortisol you released during a stressful event to clear from your body.

That means if you get angry, too hungry, or upset, it takes six hours for your body to recover.

One of the most important ways we can experience unlimited energy in our lives is by keeping our hormones balanced.

In your body, you have major hormones - as in a lot of them - and minor hormones - as in a lesser amount.

Your major hormones include:

*Cortisol and adrenalin, your stress hormones
*Insulin, the hormone that keeps your blood sugar balanced.

Your minor hormones - your progesterone, estrogen and testosterone - are all affected by your major hormones.

You can go a long way to balance your energy by keeping your cortisol, adrenalin and insulin balanced.

Why is this so important?

When you are under stress, your body experiences a phenomenon called cortisol steal. You instinctively know you don't have the energy to make a baby (the function of the sex hormones). All you can do is run away from the perceived dinosaurs!

Keeping your major hormones balanced keeps your metabolism healthy and your energy level high.

Your metabolism is defined as the sum total of the breaking down and building up processes in your body.

Your metabolism is balanced when the breaking down side - your cortisol and adrenalin - is balanced with the building up side - your insulin.

Because we are alive, we are always breaking down but whether or not we are building up depends on our lifestyle.

Cortisol is probably the most destructive substance in the body. It breaks down hair, muscle tissue, bone, even your brain chemistry.

So the equation, when it's balanced, should look like this:

Cortisol+Adrenalin = Insulin

When your hormones are not in balance, the equation really looks like this:

Cortisol+Adrenalin > Insulin

If you fail to balance the breaking down processes by building yourself up, everything breaks down and eventually you feel dried up and exhausted.

Understanding this, the question becomes, "How can I keep my major hormones balanced?"

*Daily stress management
*De-stressing energy-building exercise like yoga, tai chi and qi gong as well as walking
*Therapy to reprogram your thoughts
*Keep your blood sugar balanced by eating 5 mini meals through the day
*Avoid pro-inflammatory foods that spike your cortisol, including caffeine, alcohol, tobacco, sugar, gluten and fried foods

*Maintain a balanced rhythm of eating, work, rest and play
*Avoid high sugar junk and processed foods
*Avoid toxic emotions
*Do not over work
*Cut down on toxic chemicals, such as cigarettes, alcohol, legal and illegal drugs
*Exercise daily
*Sleep deeply at least 8 hours every night
*Go to bed by 10:30 p.m.
*Visit your doctor to test your hormone levels.

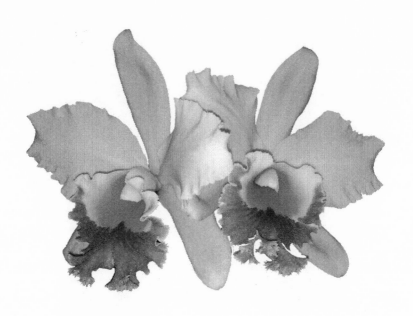

Book Two
You Could Have Danced All Night:
Your Energy Body

Chapter 1
Balancing Your Chakras

"The universe as we know it is a joint product of the observer and the observed." Pierre Teilhard de Chardin

Although you may benefit from visiting a Reiki practitioner or other energy healer, you can balance the energy centers in your body yourself, even if you never receive a Reiki attunement or learn any professional methods.

Step 1. Lie down or sit in a comfortable position.

Step 2. As you begin, say a prayer.

Dear God, I ask that you be with me right now. Please send angels, guides and protectors to balance my energy for the highest good of all. Allow me to be a clear and perfect channel for the light of your love at this time on

the planet. Thank you God, thank you God, thank you God. Amen.

Step 3. Rub your hands together to generate chi, You will feel a heat between your hands the more you rub them together - this is your own personal chi that you can use for healing.

Step 4. Place your hands on the crown of your head. Visualize and feel chi coming from your hands through the crown of your head. Hold your hands in this position until you feel your crown chakra is balanced.

Step 5. Keeping one hand on your crown chakra, move the other hand to your sixth chakra. Feel a connection between your 7th and 6th chakra. Breathe and relax, feeling and visualizing each chakra lighting up with energy.

Step 6. As you feel the connection balancing, remove the hand at the crown of your head and place both hands on your 6th chakra, balancing and opening your third eye.

Step 7. When you feel complete, take one hand and place it on your throat chakra. Feel the connection between your third eye and your throat.

Step 8. Continue on down the chakra system in this manner, taking your time and allowing yourself to feel your energy balancing. When you get to your first chakra, place both hands around your first chakra and feel your entire body relaxed, vibrant and radiating life force.

Chapter 2
Clearing Your Aura

"The law of sympathy is one of the most basic parts of magic. It states that the more similar two objects are, the greater the sympathetic link. The greater the link, the more easily they influence each other." Patrick Rothfuss

Learning how to clear your aura may be one of the easiest methods you can practice to maintain unlimited energy.

First, let's talk about what your aura actually is.

It's a law of physics that any time there is a vertical electrical current - such as exists in your body when you are standing up - there is an electrical field of energy perpendicular to that.

New age folks call that your aura.

Your energy field has been mapped by scientists and medical doctor. A healthy aura extends as much as 8 feet all around you.

Masters who practice energy exercise like yoga, tai chi and qi gong radiate auras that may extend as far as 100 feet in diameter.

You literally feel these people when they walk into a room because their energy field is so big.

As such, they can have a profound positive or negative impact because people within their periphery will resonate and harmonize with their personal vibration.

Whether your personal field is large or small, whatever is within your field has the potential to affect you - both for the good and for the worse.

Your energy field also includes the vibrations you yourself have created through your own thoughts and feelings.

When you study alternative holistic healing, you discover that illness and poor health actually begins in the energy field and comes in to the physical body.

A disturbance on the spiritual, mental, emotional or energetic layer of your field may ultimately affect you physically.

To clear your aura:

Step 1. Stand up so that you are vertical. You can do this exercise in the shower while you are also cleansing your physical body.

Step 2. Shut your eyes. Visualize the energy field that is surrounding you. You are in the center of a large circle. As you shut your eyes and look, you may see colors, you may feel energy, you may see shapes. It doesn't matter what it is, just look, feel, sense and know what is happening in your aura.

Step 3. With your eyes still shut, visualize yourself pushing the energy out away from you, through all layers of your field, out away into infinity. Breathe while you are doing this and use the power of your breath to push energy out of your field until your aura feels clear, clean and undisturbed. You will know when you are complete because you will feel calm on the inside and your field will look clear.

Step 4. Set your intention that nothing comes into your field or out of your field except unconditional love. When nothing comes in and nothing goes out except unconditional love, you will be physically and emotionally well and experience radiant prana on all levels.

Chapter 3
Clearing Your Space

"One of the basic rules of the universe is that nothing is perfect. Perfection simply doesn't exist...without imperfection, neither you nor I would exist." Stephen Hawking

The places where you live and work hold energy and emotions.

Have you ever had an argument with your spouse standing by the refrigerator?

The vibration of that fight will be left directly in that spot.

As a medical intuitive healer, I know full well that clearing your space is equally important as vacuuming, dusting and mopping.

Here are a few ways to clear any space:

1. Sage. You simply light the end of a sage stick and walk through your home, office or any other space, wafting the smoke throughout.
2. Prayer. Say a prayer in every room:

Heavenly Father, I call on the forces of nature to converge to balance all detrimental energies and increase all beneficial energies for the benefit of all living beings. I ask that this be done in the name of Jesus Christ. Amen.

3. Vortex. Visualize a vortex, the shape of a small tornado. Call on all your angels and spiritual guides. Then visualize the vortex swirling from corner to corner, clearing all detrimental vibrations. Then visualize the vortex over the actual building, pulling all detrimental energies out and up into the heavens.
4. Angels. Call on angels to position themselves at every door. I have even taken a photo with my iPhone of two angels outside my front door! Ask these angels to keep your space protected. Ask that nothing come in and nothing go out except the frequency of unconditional love.
5. Flower essences. You can muscle test which particular flower essences will balance the energy of any space. Some of my favorites are flower essence sprays from www.healingorchids.com. I particularly like Angelic Canopy, which makes you feel like you are walking into a space that is totally clear, wholesome and healthy.

6. Essential oils. You can change the frequency of any space by diffusing essential oils. Good ones to consider include rose, lavender, frankincense, sage, juniper, peppermint, basil and cedar.

7. Blue stakes. If you already know that you or your space is barraged with negativity, buy stakes at a hardware store, paint them blue and drive them into the ground around the outside corners of your home. This keeps your house's energy grounded and protected.

Chapter 4
Days of the Week

"We all have an unsuspected reserve of strength inside that emerges when life puts us to the test." Isabel Allende

One of my favorite systems of holistic alternative medicine is alchemy, a system of healing with herbs dating back to the Middle Ages. One of the earliest proponents was the nun Hildegarde von Bingen, 1098-1179.

In alchemy, they say you may have disturbances on the salt, or physical body, on the mercury, or mental/ emotional layer, or the sulfur level, which is your soul.

You could be relatively balanced on one plane but still feel uncomfortable or depleted due to an imbalance on another level.

Because you are a unique individual, each of your three aspects - your salt level, your mercury level and your sulfur level - is governed by a specific planet.

Your physical body could be ruled by one planet, your mind and emotions could be governed by another and your soul level affected by another heavenly sphere.

In alchemy, each day of the week is governed by a specific celestial body:

•**Sunday.** Planet: Sun. Color: Gold or Yellow. Chakra: Third. Scent: Ginger, Rosemary. Angel: Michael. Out of balance: Low self esteem, lack of confidence, depression and overcompensation through the ego. In balance: happy.

•**Monday.** Planet: Moon. Color: Purple. Chakra: Sixth. Scent: Jasmine, Ylang ylang. Angel: Gabriel. Out of balance: sadness, crying, moodiness, dreamy, or unrealistic. In balance: nurturing, caring, intuitive, in touch with your emotions.

•**Tuesday.** Planet: Mars. Color: Red. Chakra: Second. Scent: Pepper, Horseradish. Angel: Chamuel. Out of balance: Anger, tension, aggression, violence towards yourself or others. In balance: Bravery, courage, determination, perseverance or passion.

•**Wednesday.** Planet: Mercury. Color: Orange. Chakra: Fifth. Scent: Lavender, sage. Angel: Raphael. Out of balance: Indecisive, hyperactive, poor communication. In balance: Intelligent, adaptable, eloquent, easy going.

•**Thursday.** Planet: Jupiter. Color: Blue. Chakra: Crown. Scent: Turmeric, Cedar. Angel: Zadkiel. Out of balance: Poor judgment, over indulging, inappropriate generosity. In balance: Wise, kind, making good decisions.

•**Friday.** Planet: Venus. Color: Green. Chakra: Fourth. Scent: Rose. Angel: Haniel. Out of balance: Inappropriate or excessive love relationships, or none at all. In balance: Healthy intimate relationships, beauty and refinement.

•**Saturday.** Planet: Saturn. Color: Black. Chakra: First. Scent: Mushrooms, Asafetida. Angel: Cassiel. Out of balance: Rigid, controlling, cold, unfriendly. In balance: Detail-oriented, diplomatic, reliable, competent.

If you constantly find yourself feeling depleted on a specific day of the week, you may discover that you have a planetary imbalance.

For example, if you always feel off on Sundays, you may be experiencing a Sun imbalance, or if you are usually feeling out of kilter on Mondays, you may have a Moon imbalance.

If you find that there is a day of the week where you have a habitual imbalance, you can use kinesiology to determine whether this is due to a salt/body, mercury/mental-emotional or sulfur/soul level imbalance.

Once you know that the source is physical, mental-emotional or spiritual, you can take the actions necessary to support that specific aspect of yourself on your most depleted day.

Chapter 5
Electromagnetic Fields and Geopathic Stress

"The universe is a fractal. Whatever energy signature we carry will be repeated infinitely, again and again, until we change that vibration." Paige Bartholomew

One of the biggest sources of unexplained stress and exhaustion comes from electromagnetic fields and geopathic stress.

Electronic gadgets of all kinds produce electromagnetic fields that we can't see but which affect the electrical systems of our bodies, especially when our own chi becomes depleted.

Geopathic stress is your overall stress from your environment.

If you live in a big city, your geopathic stress may be higher than someone living in a bucolic setting. You may be exposed to:

*Cell phone towers
*Cell phones
*Microwaves
*Electric blankets
*Radio waves
*Shapes of buildings
*Waterbeds
*Radiation
*Radioactive waste
*Nuclear radiation
*Chemical runoff
*War
*Fluorescent lights
*Pagers
*TV
*Household appliances
*Airplanes
*Radar
*Satellite dishes
*Electric power lines
*Gas lines
*Coal mines
*Sick buildings
*Fumes from a new car
*Air pollution

*Water pollution
*Agricultural sprays

In addition to these obvious offenders, geopathic stress also includes natural phenomenon such as:

*Storms
*Floods
*Rivers
*Volcanic activity
*Fire
*Thunder
*Lightning
*Tidal waves
*Earthquakes
*Hurricanes
*Tsunamis
*Rainstorms
*Underground streams
*Any events on the earth, above the earth or over the earth.

Even if you are not conscious of these elements, your personal chi is directly affected by all that is around you.

Because your entire body is electrical - your heart is electrical, your brain is electrical and your energy grid is actually electrical - you may be drained by EMFs and geopathic stress more than you currently recognize.

Geopathic stress may be affecting your acupuncture meridians, chakras, organs or literally any level of your energy field.

A trained healer such as myself can identify how your body is being affected and clear the geopathic stress from your entire system.

When your personal chi is low, you may be more affected by these factors than someone whose energy field is strong and healthy.

As you build your prana, you may find yourself less reactive, but even people who are very healthy usually experience a degree of geopathic stress that they aren't consciously aware of.

You can purchase EMF protection devices from numerous sites on the internet.

Because you are vibrationally unique, no one device will work for everybody. You can use kinesiology to determine which protection method will work best to keep you centered in your own energy.

Chapter 6
Five Flows of Breath

"As you breathe in, cherish yourself. As you breathe out, cherish all beings." The 14th Dalai Lama

One of the most important ways to experience unlimited energy open is to open your five flows of breath.

At an atomic level, your body is 65 percent oxygen. http://en.wikipedia.org/wiki/Composition_of_the_ human_body

Just because you are alive doesn't mean that you are breathing optimally.

In yoga, we say that there are five flows, called vayus, of your breath:

1. Your inhale. Prana vayu.
2. Your exhale. Apana vayu.
3. Your breath around your waist. Samana vayu.

4. Your breath around your head. Udana vayu.
5. The breath radiating from your navel into your arms, legs and head governing whole-body circulation. Vyana vayu.

Often what happens is that one of the five flows of breath shuts down.

You can use kinesiology to muscle test if all five flows are working for you.

For example, the most common phenomenon that I see is people with high blood pressure who do not exhale properly.

If you hook up a person with high blood pressure to a monitor that reads their EKG, you will see that they inhale and then nothing really seems to happen with their exhale.

You can heal high blood pressure completely just by learning to breathe fully and learning how to exhale.

Here is a simple technique to open all five flows of your breath for greater vitality.

I call this Eight Minutes to Inner Peace:

Start by sitting or lying down in a comfortable position.

1. *One Minute*: Focus on lengthening your inhale.
2. *One Minute*: Focus on lengthening your exhale.
3. *One Minute*: Focus on making your inhale and exhale equally long and deep.

If you have been lying down, sit up for the next five breathing techniques.

4. *One Minute*: Bellows Breath. Inhale into your belly and exhale forcibly by contracting your solar plexus.

5. *One Minute*: Breath of Fire. Inhaling and exhaling rapidly, pump your diaphragm. Your inhale will happen naturally.

6. *One Minute*: Alternate nostril breathing. Inhale through your right nostril. With the thumb of your right hand, close the right nostril. Exhale through your left nostril. With the ring finger of your right hand, close the left nostril. Exhale through your right nostril. Use your thumb to close your right nostril. Exhale through the left nostril. Use your ring finger to close the left. Repeat.

7. *One Minute*: Bumblebee breath. Place your pointer finger and middle finger on your forehead. Place your thumbs on your ear flaps and close your ears. Place your ring finger lightly on your closed eyelids. Little finger rests on your cheekbones. Make a humming sound like a bee.

8. *One Minute*: Ocean breath. Open your mouth, relax your jaw. Inhale and make the sound of the ocean in the back of your throat. Exhale and make the sound of the ocean. Close your lips and continue making the sound of the ocean.

If you would like to watch a video of each of these breathing exercises for greater clarification, please visit: http://unlimitedenergynow.com/eight-minutes-to-inner-peace-breathing-exercises-pranayama/.

Chapter 7
Grounding

"Everything we do is infused with the energy with which we do it. If we're frantic, life will be frantic. If we're peaceful, life will be peaceful." Marianne Williamson

Those of us who are gardeners know and experience the tremendous chi that we feel when we connect to the earth.

The frequency of the earth is 7.83 HZ.

HZ is a symbol for hertz, a measure of frequency. 1 HZ is one cycle per second.

When you spend time connecting to the earth, your whole body comes into resonance with this frequency, which has surprisingly dramatic healing benefits, restoring your natural circadian rhythm on all levels.

Our brain may naturally produce alpha brain waves - the brain waves at 8 to 12 HZ that help us relax - when we are connected to the 7.83 HZ of the earth.

When we are awake and alert, we are in a beta brain-wave state, 13 to 30 HZ.

It is a well-known scientific fact that your brain must produce alpha brain waves - the brain waves just below beta - in order for true relaxation to occur.

When you finally relax, the production of your stress hormones stops and actual healing occurs.

Some scientists have even speculated that 7.83 HZ is the precise frequency at which DNA repairs.

Cell phones, power lines, microwaves and other potentially harmful electromagnetic frequencies occur at much higher frequency hertz, keeping us in a state of undetected stress.

Dirt may not seem like all that much to those who see it from afar, but watch what happens when you walk barefoot when the weather allows.

As we ground, we experience our bodies more fully, allow our feelings and connect with our true self in a healthy way.

When we are ungrounded, we often make poor choices.

We over exercise, over work, drink too much, eat too much and don't notice how we or other people feel when we say or do the wrong things.

Grounding ourselves in our bodies and connecting to the earth quietly empowers us to be in the present moment where all joy actually occurs.

Because earth is yin, being connected to earth is a great way to balance your own personal yin chi.

Yin energy is dark, of the earth, quiet and still.

Yang energy is light, full of movement and activity.

Our society tends to be too yang.

Too much yang activity tends to lead to chronic illnesses like fatigue, fibromyalgia, and cancer.

When you have been so yang throughout your life that your yin energy is out of balance, you can rebalance yourself by grounding.

Here are a few simple ways you can ground your energy:

*Garden
*Walk barefoot
*Take your shoes off inside your home
*Call your spirit back to your body
*Take time to feel all your feelings
*Care for plants inside your home or office
*Turn off your computers, the internet, cell phones and TV
*Walk outside in nature
*Beat a drum
*Dance
*Take a shower
*Clean your house

*Vacuum or wash your floors
*Listen to your own heart beat
*Listen to the sound of the rain
*Do nothing

As you ground yourself in the here and the now, you will find yourself deeply restored.

Chapter 8
Healing Your Hara Line

"I am not what happened to me, I am what I choose to become." Carl Jung

Because your hara line is an important conduit for unlimited energy in your body, it is helpful to take steps every day to heal your hara.

What is your hara?

Your hara is the vertical line of electrical current running from the earth through your body all the way through the crown of your head up to the divine universal source.

When your hara is open and clear, you experience unlimited energy.

When there is a block, congestion or blow out in this vertical current, you may feel exhausted without knowing how to make yourself feel better.

Here is how to keep this essential personal power line clear:

Step 1. Lying or sitting, get comfortable.

Step 2. Imagine that your energy body has floated perpendicular out of your physical body in front of you.

Step 3. In your mind's eye, see your energy body between the palms of your two hands. Visualize your hara line smaller and shorter - about 12 inches - between the palms of your hands stretched out in front of you.

Step 4. Visualize your left hand above the crown of your head. Imagine your right hand below your feet. With your left hand, begin to sweep through your energy field from your feet to the crown of your head. See yourself removing any energy blockages in your hara line. You may feel subtle blips of vibration. You may see holes or blow outs in your hara. Whatever you perceive, affirm that your right hand has the power to remove, release and heal all the energy blockages that you discover.

Step 5. As you sweep your left hand from right to left, visualize a bright white light sending healing chi into your hara. Repeat three or four times until your hara line feels open and clear. As you are sweeping your right hand through your hara and radiating the bright light of healing, use an invocation:

I invoke the light of the Christ within.
I am a clear and perfect channel.
Love and light are my guides.

Step 6. After your hara line feels completely clear, hold your two hands in front of you, visualizing once again your left hand above the crown of your head and your right hand below your feet. Use an affirmation:

I am a clear and perfect channel.
I am a channel of light and love.
Today I channel the highest vibration possible.
Thank you God, thank you all my angels.
I am guided and protected.
Amen. It is done.

Step 7. Now visualize your hara line back in your physical body. Feel your energy flowing easily from the divine above you down into the center of the earth below you.

Chapter 9
Over Energy Versus Under Energy

"The atoms or elementary particles themselves are not real; they form a world of potentialities or possibilities rather than one of things or facts." Werner Heisenberg

If I am doing a medical intuitive reading, what I will literally do is read the life force in your organs, acupuncture meridians, chakras and overall body.

A healthy functioning organ, meridian, chakra or body will often be operating between 72 and 85 percent.

Many people who are overachievers want to be an A+ student. However, often we can experience difficulties when organs, muscles, meridians or chakras are over working.

Over working tends to lead to under energy.

Under energy is what I see when I am looking at chronic fatigue, fibromyalgia and other long-term illnesses. Laid back individuals generally do not develop chronic fatigue.

The long-term pattern of overdoing leads to depletion. You are truly only as resilient as your weakest organ.

Your body may look great on the outside through over exercising, for example, but if you suddenly experience a heart attack because you have depleted yourself, looking good won't get you too far.

Often it feels good - initially - to do the wrong things because you feel high from the initial rush of adrenalin. Stay up all night. Skip meals. Go on high speed chases.

Instead of over energy or under energy in any area, what you want to experience is balance.

If you are experiencing a chronic illness, you may have not understood this concept and depleted yourself to the point of sickness and fatigue.

Chapter 10
Protection Rituals

"Trust the vibes you get, energy doesn't lie." Shan Harlin

Even though it's all one unlimited energy, and it's all good, within that one energy there are numerous frequencies, not all of which feel pleasant to experience.

If you live in an urban area, like New York, London or Atlanta, the combined negativity may include frequencies that drag you down.

There is much less negativity at the beach, in the open land or mountains, but it's still present everywhere to some degree.

One of the ways you can keep yourself centered and grounded is to learn how to protect your personal frequency.

What you need to do to protect your field may be unique to you. Different methods work better for different people. Here are a few good ones:

1. Do not wear black clothing. The color black attracts negativity. I never wear black when I am doing healing work.

2. Wear purple bracelets around your wrists. The color purple cuts off negativity. If you do any work that involves putting your hands on people, please wear purple around your wrists.

3. Wear white. The color white deflects negativity.

4. Snowflake obsidian, smokey quartz, black tourmaline, laboradite, amethyst, Apache tear, bloodstone, green tourmaline, amber, azeztulite and citrine stones may be used for this purpose.

5. Visualize yourself inside a bubble. On the outside, visualize the color silver like a mirror reflecting negativity. On the inside, visualize the color gold, the highest frequency of the aura.

6. Affirm: "I have nothing to give or receive except unconditional love."

7. Take a bath with one cup Epsom salts to one cup baking soda. This formula clears your aura and allows you to release any negativity at the end of the day.

8. Say a prayer asking God, your angels and all your spiritual guides to keep you centered, grounded and protected throughout the day.

9. Flower essences. I recommend Soul Shield+ by www.healingorchids.com or Fringed Violet from www.ausflowers.com.au.

10. Visualize a screen over your third chakra. People who are high in the psychic gift of feeling tend to pick up the energy of other people's emotions. If you can think of a door with a metal fly screen, visualize a fly screen over your third chakra.

Chapter 11

Rhythm

"You had the power all along, my dear." Glenda, The Good Witch, Wizard of Oz

You can enjoy vibrant chi by establishing a consistent healthy rhythm in your daily life.

Different organs and meridians are active at specific times of day.

5 to 7 a.m.: **Large intestine** time. Drink water first thing. Move your bowels.

7 to 9 a.m.: **Stomach** time. Eat breakfast, the most important meal of your day.

9 to 11 a.m.: **Pancreas.** Enzymes from your pancreas process what you have just eaten.

11 a.m. to 1 p.m.: **Heart.** Your heart pumps blood through your body.

1 to 3 p.m.: **Small intestine.** Your small intestine assimilates nutrients from the food you have eaten.

3 to 5 p.m.: **Bladder.** Your bladder clears.

5 to 7 p.m.: **Kidney** time. Your kidney filters your blood.

7 to 9 p.m.: **Circulation** time. Your body circulates nutrients into your cells.

9 to 11 p.m.: **Triple warmer** time. Your endocrine system resets.

11 p.m. to 1 p.m.: **Gall bladder.** Your gall bladder cleanses your tissues.

1 to 3 a.m.: **Liver.** Your liver detoxifies.

3 to 5 a.m.: **Lung.** You inhale and exhale while sleeping deeply.

By understanding the natural flow of prana through our meridians, we can identify which organs or meridians are out of balance if we consistently experience low points at specific times of day.

For example, if you are constantly exhausted from 1 to 3 p.m., you may need to support your small intestine by taking digestive enzymes with your lunch and giving yourself time to process your meal afterwards.

If you do not live in harmony with your personal rhythm, you may find yourself feeling exhausted even if there is nothing wrong with your job, your kids, your marriage or anything else in your life.

Chapter 12
The Five Elements

"The more you lose yourself in something bigger than yourself, the more energy you will have." Norman Vincent Peale

In order to have good chi, you have to balance the five elements inside yourself.

The five element theory comes from Chinese medicine.

When you understand the five elements, you can learn what naturally builds your chi and what destroys it.

Fire element includes the acupuncture meridians for your heart, small intestines, triple warmer and heart protector. It is represented by the color red.

Earth element includes the acupuncture meridians for your stomach and spleen. It is represented by yellow.

Metal element includes the acupuncture meridians for your lungs and large intestine. It is represented by the color white.

Water element includes the acupuncture meridians for your kidneys and bladder. It is represented by the color blue.

Wood element includes the acupuncture meridians for your liver and gallbladder. It is represented by the color green.

In Chinese medicine, the Creation cycle describes one flow of energy. Fire creates earth. Earth creates metal. Metal creates water. Water creates wood. Wood creates fire.

In the Control cycle, water controls fire. Fire controls metal. Metal controls wood. Wood controls earth. Earth controls water.

Often, when we feel exhausted, we can reflect on our five elements to discover where we are out of balance.

For example, too much fire energy - too much passion - puts out our water energy and depletes our kidney chi.

We can bring the five elements into balance in ourselves by healing the underlying organs, through our diet and by placing more attention on the organs that are depleted.

Chapter 13
Your Energy Score Sheet

"We either make ourselves miserable or we make ourselves strong. The amount of work is the same."
Carlos Castaneda

Even if you don't know anything about chi or prana, you can usually tell what makes you feel more alive and what exhausts you.

On two separate sheets of paper, write down exactly what strengthens your inner light.

Energy boosters may include:

*Meditation
*Taking a hot bath
*Playing with your kids
*Going to lunch with a friend

*Being in nature
*Gardening
*Enjoying your hobbies
*Going on vacation
*Laughing
*Visiting a comedy club
*Drinking water
*Receiving massage
*Sitting quietly
*Taking a nap
*Practicing yoga, tai chi or qi gong
*Going to a party
*Spending a quiet evening by yourself
*Walking your dog
*Listening to poetry
*Going to a concert
*Learning something new and exciting
*Cleaning your house
*Wearing crystal gemstones
*Taking an Epsom salt bath
*Drinking tea
*Dancing
*Breath work
*Going home from work on time
*Travel
*Meeting new people
*Writing in your journal
*Challenging yourself at work
*Watching football

*Playing a game
*Alternating hot and cold water in the shower
*Self massage, stimulating all your neurolymphatic points
*Saying I am sorry and meaning it
*Playing the drums or a musical instrument of your choice
*Walking to the top of a mountain and enjoying the view
*Wrapping yourself in a warm blanket
*Taking one afternoon off every week if you are able
*Praying
*Writing a list of intentions every week
*Reading spiritual books
*Joining a spiritual community
*Forming a spiritual family of like-minded friends
*Unplugging from the computer
*Going for a walk
*Taking 5 to 10 minute breaks during your work day
*Doing "stealth exercise," taking short walks up the stairs at work
*Listening to your angels
*Taking one day off every week to rest and do nothing
*Gardening
*Raising orchids, the most evolved flowers on the face of the earth
*Daily exercise
*Drinking enough water
*Making a healthy meal for your family
*Raising your own vegetable garden
*Looking up old friends

*Challenging yourself to do something you have never done before
*Losing weight
*Giving up junk food
*Doing something good for others with no expectation of being rewarded
*Sharing your own abundance with people who need it
*Random acts of kindness
*Carrying food for the homeless in your car, such as little packs of nuts
*Being consistent with your schedule
*Going to bed on time
*Looking your best
*Figuring out what makes you happy

Energy Robbers May Include:

*Fighting or arguing
*Staying up late
*Drinking coffee after 5 pm
*Eating junk food
*Eating microwaved food
*Being dehydrated
*Drinking too much alcohol
*Smoking
*Overworking
*Over exercising
*Being around unpleasant people
*Holding grudges

*Not cleaning up your clutter
*Wearing old clothes that no longer fit
*Surrounding yourself with objects that bring up unpleasant memories
*Not getting enough sleep
*Not taking time for yourself
*Exercise where your heart rate is constantly over 100 beats per minute or more, such as running, jogging, spinning classes, triathlons or boot camps
*Not exercising at all
*Failing to recognize your own needs
*Placing others ahead of yourself at all times
*Not recognizing that you are important
*Anger
*Grief
*Pride
*Fear
*Shame
*Blame
*Apathy
*Cravings and addictions
*Depression
*Anxiety
*Withdrawal from loved ones

As you make your own list of what restores your life force and what depletes it, notice where you spend most of your time.

Are you spending more of your time with people and activities that build your chi? Or are you spending most of your time with people, situations and activities that use up your personal vitality? You can begin to balance your energy equation by noticing what revitalizes you and what drains you.

Chapter 14
Your Energy System

"People inspire you or they drain you - pick them wisely."
Hans F. Hansen

In order to experience unlimited energy you will want to understand your personal energy system.

There's a natural flow to this energy system:

1. Energy enters through a point on the crown of your head called the Ba hui.
2. Through this point, energy channels through your hara line, a vertical electrical current going down into the center of the earth and all the way up into the heavens.
3. Your hara line feeds energy into your chakras.
4. Your chakras feed energy into your acupuncture system.

5. Your acupuncture meridians feed energy into your organs.
6. Your organs feed energy into your muscles.

Once you understand this flow, you may be able to figure out where the problem is by thinking in reverse.

If you have problem with a particular muscle, for example, you may be having difficulty with the organ that muscle is related to.

Every muscle in your body is related to a specific organ, a specific acupuncture meridian and a specific chakra.

Muscles related to organ systems and meridians:

Your hamstrings and fascia latae are related to your large intestine.

Your pectoralis major clavicular and neck muscles are related to your stomach.

Your latissimus dorsi is related to your spleen.

Your subscapularis is related to your heart.

Your quadriceps are related to your small intestine.

Your peroneus is related to your bladder.

Your psoas is related to your kidneys.

Your gluteus medius is related to your circulation.

Your teres minor is related to your triple warmer.

Your anterior deltoid is related to your gallbladder.

Your pectoralis major sternal is related to your liver.

Your anterior serratus is related to your lungs.

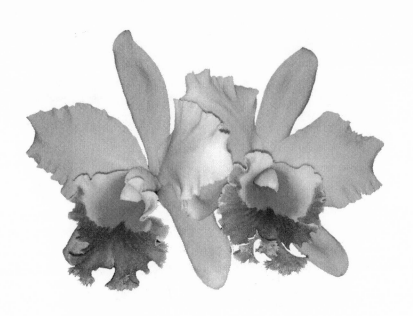

Book Three
The Big High That Never Ends:
Your Emotional Body

Chapter 1

Acting Your Age

"One small crack does not mean that you are broken, it means that you were put to the test and you didn't fall apart." Linda Poindexter

If you stay in the consciousness of your present age, more than likely, if you are reading this book, you have developed some degree of wisdom.

Life teaches us and seasons us to develop the spiritual strength to persevere.

However, on an emotional level, we often get triggered by people, places or events. When we get triggered, we often revert emotionally to an earlier age where more than likely a trauma occurred.

One of the important steps you can take to experience unlimited energy is to find out what age you act when:

*You spell words
*You go out on a date
*You cook a meal
*You deal with money
*You get into an argument
*You look for a job
*You eat a meal
*You find yourself feeling stressed

When people, places or events pull up an earlier aspect of ourselves, we temporarily lose our wisdom chi.

Let me give you a perfect example.

There's an old saying, "If you think you are enlightened, go spend a week with your family."

How old do you really act when you are around your family of origin?

Here's a simple way to find out:

1. You probably already know your current chronological age. Have a friend use kinesiology to muscle test your current overall emotional age. If you are 40 years old chronologically you could theoretically actually be older emotionally provided you have developed your wisdom self. If your emotional age is actually younger, you will want to do emotional processing to clear out your baggage.
2. Once you know your chronological and emotional age, check how old you act in the above situations. If you

are constantly reverting to an earlier age, you are also dropping your chi every time you regress.

3. If you recognize, for example, that you do not act your age when you deal with money or when you sit down to eat, ask your mind, body and soul what you need to do to maintain your present wisdom age in those situations.

The more you can stay in the present moment in all situations, the more you will experience unlimited energy.

Chapter 2

Allowing Your Emotions to Flow

"It takes the same amount of energy to worry as it does to believe." Joel Osteen

One of the patterns that keeps you feeling perpetually sick and tired is the habit of trying to keep a lid on all your emotions.

E-motions are just energy in motion.

When we feel whatever it is that we are feeling, we allow the energy to flow.

It takes a tremendous amount of chi to try to stop the flow of our feelings. When we repress or suppress what we are feeling, that leaves us totally exhausted.

One of the best ways to create a safe space to feel your emotions is with what I call The Container Exercise:

1. If and when you feel your emotions coming up and you feel in any way overwhelmed by the intensity of what you are feeling, begin by imagining a container.

2. Your container could be very very small, such as a dainty little teacup, or very very big, such as a dumpster.

3. Once you have created the container in your mind, allow yourself to feel all your feelings until the container is filled up. Breathe into whatever you are feeling and explore your feelings with all your senses. See them. Feel them. Hear them. Know what it's all about.

4. Once your container is now full, visualize yourself emptying your container. You could visualize yourself throwing the contents of the teacup out the window. You could imagine the City Sanitation Department coming along and picking up the dumpster. Either way, get rid of it.

5. Now shift your vibration. Get up from where ever you were and go and do something different. Give yourself permission to shift your focus. Change your energy channel!

What's so great about the container exercise?

1. It allows you to feel safe while you are feeling all your emotions.

2. It creates boundaries so you will know that there is a beginning and end for the time being.

3. It empowers you with a feeling of control, so that you don't feel overtaken by the severity of what you are feeling.
4. It gives you permission to process your emotions at your own pace.

In my practice, I have worked with clients with every kind of addiction you could possibly imagine: alcoholics, workaholics, foodaholics, exercise bulimics, prescription drug addicts, people who are addicted to illegal drugs. And that's for starters.

The common denominator in all these patterns I find is that addictions are just a handy way to avoid our feelings.

I tell my clients you will know you are well when you can finally get angry, have a panic attack or feel lonely and sad and cry without having to take a drink, work 14 hours, overeat, over exercise or take a pill.

You can say to yourself, "*I am safe. This is only my feelings!*"

You know you are very strong when you are strong enough to handle your emotions, knowing that whatever you are feeling in this moment is just energy that will flow through you and pass.

Giving yourself permission to let the air out of your emotions may also be one of the simplest natural healing remedies you have ever tried to overcome chronic fatigue.

Because it takes so much energy to hold back the waves of our emotions, you may not have had any idea how much you exhaust yourself through the habit of suppressing and repressing your feelings.

Benefits of allowing your emotions to flow include increased vitality and decreased pain.

You may be shocked how you can get rid of every manner of discomfort and dis-ease simply by feeling whatever it is that is going on inside yourself.

Chapter 3
Choose Not To Suffer

"Once you believe in yourself and see your soul as divine and precious, you'll automatically be converted to a being who can create miracles." Wayne Dyer

As they say, pain is inevitable, suffering is optional.

A lot of people are not aware of the difference between pain and suffering, but they are as different, though completely related, as night and day.   Pain is our physical experience. It's the stub in the toe, the ache in the side, the head pounding, the muscle grabbing, the nerve shooting.

Suffering is our mental emotional experience of the pain. It's the story we tell ourselves about how awful everything is. The louder we complain, the more we reinforce our right to feel bad.

Both pain and suffering drag down your vitality terribly. When we choose to lessen the suffering, even if there is still pain, we can maintain more of our personal life force.

When we experience pain, one way to choose not to suffer is to refuse to put words onto it.

Our immediate instinct is to put a story onto the pain. "He/she made me do it," the story begins. The underlying message is, "I am a victim," whether it's a victim even of just the pain.

You are a being of unlimited power and potential.

When you suffer a pain, immediately go into the feeling of it.

Literally feel the vibration.

When you feel the energy of an event, you immediately allow the prana to flow and that gives the chi some place to go and it begins to release.

On the other hand, if you resist the experience, your pain and suffering will most likely intensify and your personal energy will continue to drop.

Chapter 4

Emotional Blockages Deplete Your Chi Faster Than Anything

"Energy is a state of mind. Tell yourself you're tired and you will be. Tell yourself you feel great and you will." Charlene Johnson

Many of my clients who are eating well, exercising right and taking other wonderful steps to feel good often still find themselves drained with nothing to spare at the end of the day.

Unresolved emotional issues deplete your chi faster than junk good, a bad night's sleep or most anything you could think of.

Why is this case?

If you understand the human energy system, our emotional layer is actually the largest part of us.

Emotions can shut down literally any physiological process.

Think of the stories of women fainting at the announcement of bad news.

Notice how your own tears swell up when you learn of a personal tragedy.

Resentment, bitterness, grudges, old hurts, all these deplete your chi, block your organ flow, weaken your acupuncture meridians, decrease your breath, interrupt your thoughts and weigh down your soul.

Understanding this fact, it's essential to do core healing emotional work if you find yourself constantly depleted.

Taking care of yourself emotionally is equally important as eating well or exercising regularly.

According to Dr. David Hawkins, M.D., author of *Power Vs. Force,* every emotion you feel has a level of consciousness associated with it.

Our emergency emotions can be summarized:

Pride
Anger
Desire
Fear
Grief
Apathy
Guilt
Shame

The lower your emotional tone, the more exhausted you will more likely feel.

If you find yourself feeling exhausted, tune in to what you are feeling and discover the underlying emotional drain.

Chapter 5
Gratitude

"Gratitude energy generates an astonishing power of feelings within us." Marcella Zinner

You can't feel grateful and depressed at the same time.

If you want to experience unlimited energy right now, FEEL grateful.

Many of us can rattle off a list of blessings: family and friends, perhaps a house, a job or maybe a bit of money.

It's one thing to think about a blessing.

It's quite another to shift your vibration totally by FEELING thankful - really allowing the awareness to shift into a whole-body sensation.

Feeling grateful puts you in the frequency of love and appreciation, which allows your spirit to soar.

When we feel grateful as opposed to merely thinking in our heads about what we are grateful for, energetically our hearts open and our minds quiet.

How do you start?

Make a gratitude list.

Now, as you look at your list, feel the whole-body sensations that arise as you ponder each blessing.

Allow the energy of each gift to flow through you. Notice where in your body you feel the frequency. Most likely you will feel this frequency in your heart.

Chapter 6
Pleasure

"To give pleasure to a single heart by a single act is better than a thousand heads bowing in prayer." Mahatma Gandhi

One of the ways to be truly happy in life is through the avenue of our physical body.

Eating delicious food. Enjoying sex. Feeling the sunshine on your skin, the water flowing over your back as you go for a swim or take a shower. Hugging and being hugged.

Taking the time to enjoy physical pleasure is one of the most important avenues for restoring your energy.

Many people feel that they ought to be working, saving the planet, tending their children or making money rather than having fun and enjoying themselves.

However, if you live such a driven life that you fail to allow yourself physical pleasure, you may experience less vitality and find it much more difficult to do the things you need to do.

It's all about balance.

Qi gong and tai chi masters talk about your jing, which is energy you were naturally born with that gets stored in your kidneys.

Depending on whether you are a man or a woman, your jing creates your sperm or eggs. Having a healthy sex drive is a sign of good chi both in men and in women.

Many people shut down energetically or emotionally over this issue due to poor programming or unresolved issues from our past.

We need to understand that hormones drive behavior.

For example, if your insulin is out of balance, you may feel hungry all the time.

When we have healthy testosterone levels, we need to have a sexual release, whether we are a man or a woman.

When we honor and allow all aspects of ourselves - the physical animal as well as our spiritual self - we can enjoy unlimited energy in every aspect of our lives.

Chapter 7
The Emotions That Make You Sick

"Every experience, no matter how bad it seems, holds within it a blessing of some kind. The goal is to find it."
Buddha

If you study holistic alternative medicine, you will discover that literally every disease has a specific vibration and a specific emotion attached to it.

It's my experience that you can't actually clear any illness unless you also release the emotions that caused it.

When you understand the correlation between clearing your emotions - not just talking about them or even understanding them but actually moving beyond them - and your unlimited energy, you will want to take the steps necessary to stay emotionally clear.

How do you do that?

Step 1. Each time you experience an illness, disease or suffer from an accident, take the time to ask your body what message you need to hear.

Step 2. Find the emotion attached to the illness, disease or accident. Maybe you were feeling a certain way when you got sick or suffered the trauma.

Step 3. What would you need to do in order to let go of the emotion? If you did let go of that feeling, how would your life be different?

Step 4. Visualize a picture of what you would look like if you let go of that emotion. Ask yourself what you hear if you let go of that feeling. And finally, ask yourself how you would feel if you let it all go.

Step 5. If you need outside support to let go, set up an appointment with a body worker, therapist or alternative healer. As you process your emotions more easily, notice how you your unlimited energy returns.

Chapter 8
What You Really Need To Be Happy

"The higher your energy level, the more efficient your body. The more efficient your body, the better you feel and the more you will use your talent to produce outstanding results." Anthony Robbins

One of the most profound ways to experience unlimited energy is by being totally honest with yourself about what you actually need to be truly happy.

Many times in life, we operate by other people's standards.

We are told to go to certain schools, enter certain professions, live in a certain way but that's not what our true self is actually longing to do.

You are here to do you - not anybody else.

Your true soul gift is to give your specific vibration in the way that you alone can contribute.

Give yourself permission to follow your soul's true longing and you will find yourself uncovering vitality you never even realized that you had!

What do you really need to be happy in your life right now?

Check off which ones apply to you:

I need to be physically fit.
I need to own beautiful clothes.
I need to have a soul mate.
I need to run my own business.
I need to retire.
I need to be organized.
I need a clean house.
I need time in nature.
I need time to exercise every day.
I need time with my family.
I need close friends.
I need to travel.
I need to contribute to the lives of others.
I need to laugh.
I need to perform.
I need special recognition from others.
I need time alone.
I need more time to be with others.
I need to have a child.
I need to experience true inner peace.

I need to make more money.
I need to be financially secure.
I need to be a boss.
I need to work in a group.
I need to work by myself.
I need to create works of art.
I need a hobby.
I need to feel safe.
I need to listen to my angels.
I need to cook delicious meals.
I need to own my home.
I need to live in a different country.
I need to take care of the environment.
I need to heal others.
I need to be with animals.
I need to study and learn.
I need to be a saver.
I need to play a musical instrument.
I need to work at home.
I need to travel for my work.
I need to teach others.
I need to tend a garden.
I need rest.
I need meditation.
I need to have large family gatherings.
I need to take care of children.
I need my financial affairs in order.
I need to experience a new way of living.
I need a new partner.

I need to express my sacred sexuality.
I need to be hugged.
I need to give and receive gifts.
I need to love and be loved.
I need romance.
I need to be listened to.

As you listen to the wisdom of your soul, you are naturally led to what makes you really happy. Have the courage to follow this wisdom.

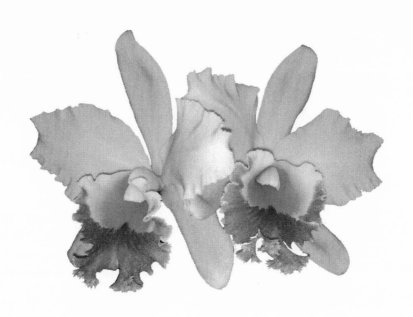

Book Four
Unleash Your Inner Genius:
Your Mental Body

Chapter 1

Always Look For the Best Possible Thought

"Everything is energy and that's all there is to it. Match the frequency of the reality you want and you cannot help but get that reality. It can be no other way. This is not philosophy. This is physics." Albert Einstein

If your car breaks down by the side of the road, you may not initially feel like jumping for joy.

But when you make an effort to look for the best possible thought, you may soon have a great day regardless because you shifted the vibration behind any given event.

It may feel very personal when your car breaks down in the pouring rain, when your spouse walks out and asks for divorce, when the kids leave home and immediately get into trouble, but the truth is that we are all just souls having a human experience and that human experience usually includes a few surprises along the way.

When we let go of the habit of judging the surprises that come our way, we can go more easily with the flow, allowing our frequency and attention to shift.

How do you always look for the best possible thought?

1. Have a fool-proof positive thought - a thought so inspiring that it lights up your heart no matter when you think of it. You could visualize yourself hugging your dog, dancing in the moonlight or holding the hand of your mate. Feel the energy and allow your vibration to shift.
2. In any given situation, bless all that happens. You may not immediately know why just yet, but affirm that you have been blessed. Bless everyone around you too.
3. See the humor and have a laugh.
4. If you find yourself wallowing in negativity, change the channel. Just as you would change the channel if you were surfing through TV programs and landed on a show you didn't want to watch, notice when your energy drops and do something different. Go for a walk. Call a friend. Read a good book. Sing a song. Say a prayer. Meditate.

Chapter 2
Ask and Ye Shall Receive

"The problem is not the problem; the problem is your attitude about the problem." Captain Jack Sparrow

Every organ, every muscle and every endocrine gland holds the energy of specific emotions.

The emotion behind your adrenal gland is will.

Many people literally exhaust themselves by using their willpower to drive everything - not only their own lives, but the lives of everybody around them - even the weather!

Focusing your mind on specific goals, you can override your deeper feelings, over power your fears, your reservations and self doubt, disregard your body's intelligence and make goals happen no matter what.

Although you may get things done, the habit of pushing and shoving yourself through your willpower can exhaust you and possibly everybody around you literally on all levels.

If you think life has to be a certain perfect way - just so - in order to be acceptable in your eyes, you are probably quite tired as this is not the way life energy actually unfolds.

We think life should move in a straight line, following the ego's directives with no side detours, but all living energy - the galaxies, hurricanes, even the petals of a sunflower - moves in a spiral pattern.

The spiral of life keeps us from totally seeing the surprises just ahead around the corner.

How do you get things done without exhaustion?

The Bible directs "Ask and ye shall receive."

If there is something you really want in your life, say a prayer.

Ask specifically, "Dear God, please bless me with this OR something better."

You allow the possibility that although you may think you know the best possible outcome, our ego minds in fact do not possess all possible information.

This prayer comes from a humble but wise mind.

The truth is that the unlimited energy of all that is, Universal God Source, has its own intelligence.

Often we think we know the ideal outcome in any given situation.

When we allow the mystery of life to unfold, we often give thanks for our unanswered prayers!

When we allow that something better may in fact be the best of all possibilities, we open ourselves to the truth of life, that our ego minds are in fact quite limited and that often our soul knows best.

Chapter 3
Discover Where You Give Your Power Away

"When you find peace within yourself, you become the kind of person who can live at peace with others." Peace Pilgrim

You are an unlimited being with far more power and potential than you may possibly even realize.

Nevertheless, many of us have bought into the idea that we have limitations.

We think we aren't good enough.

This is such a universal dilemma, virtually every human should receive a healing to let go of the core belief that you aren't good enough.

You may think you aren't tall enough, rich enough, good looking enough, well dressed enough, educated enough, pretty enough, thin enough, smart enough or have enough.

All these thoughts about our perceived lack and limitations sink our life force like a heavy stone.

There are two ways you may have developed these crazy ideas:

1. Buy in. When you buy in, that means that someone long ago told you that you were inherently imperfect. Because our minds are so impressionable when we are young, these limiting beliefs may have been instilled by your parents. In turn, your parents were programmed by their parents because in fact nobody actually knew any better.

2. Sell out. When you sell out, you let go of your own personal convictions and you go along for convenience with the prevailing beliefs, no matter how unhealthy or irrational or unhelpful they may be. You accept the idea that there is a recession/depression in the economy, so you participate in that party rather than participating in your own recovery. You go along with the junk food that's presented to you, rather than reaching for food that is actually healthy.

If you discover that you have bought in or sold out, set your intention to take your power back.

Do not allow other people to determine your own reality.

Do not allow other people's negative projections to determine your emotional state, your financial state, your social state or any other important aspect of your life.

Once you recognize to whom you have given your power away, you can follow this self healing process:

Step 1. Visualize your mother, father or other people whose ideas you have bought into or sold out to. It could be the mass media telling you what they think the condition of the world is. That may be true for others, but it doesn't have to be true for you.

Step 2. In your mind, tell your mother, father or other people or organizations that you forgive them. You know that by saying to you whatever they did, they were in fact just looking out for what they thought were your best interests. On a soul level even, they are all here for your highest good.

Say silently or out loud:

Father/Mother/People/Organization:

I forgive you.

Thank you for the blessing of your good intentions.

I now take my power back and give myself permission to create and experience my own truth.

I love you.

I know you love me.

Thank you thank you thank you.

I now live by my word and my truth, acting for the highest good of all from my own best intentions in my own power.

Amen.

Chapter 4

Don't Let Anyone Else Drink Your Milkshake

"Give yourself permission to immediately walk away from anything that gives you bad vibes. There is no need to explain or make sense of it. Just trust what you feel."
Sonia Choquette

If you work in a corporate job, you may be prone to working longer hours than you are actually paid for.

In many cases, this is expected as par for the course.

However, when you continue to work longer hours than you are actually paid for, you are allowing someone else to drink your milkshake.

You literally give away your life energy - your wisdom, your youth and your vitality - to benefit the corporation.

Often, when we are starting out in our careers, we need to learn certain skills in order to succeed.

If you allow other people to drink your milkshake early on, that may be O.K. for awhile, but if you continue to be paid for 40 hours a week and actually work 50, 60, 70, or 80 hours for somebody else, you develop an energy imbalance.

If this is happening, make a choice.

Either continue to work in an environment where you allow a corporation to suck the life out of you or gather the essential skills you need to strike out on your own.

If you work extra hours to develop the mastery to one day become your own boss, you can think of it almost like an apprentice program where you are being paid a lower wage in order to learn.

But once you have gathered the knowledge and experience you need, cut yourself loose and give yourself permission to use your life force for your own benefit, for your own higher purposes.

Chapter 5

Gamesmanship

"You have to learn the rules of the game. And then you have to play better than anyone else." Albert Einstein

One of the easiest ways to shift your frequency is to start treating your life as a game.

Too many of us take our lives as if everything were a matter of life or death: the fourth quarter report of a large corporation, our children's grades in school, whether or not we get a raise, promotion or better job, how much we weigh on a scale, what's happening to the world economy.

It's enough to make you feel like you would rather have stayed in bed!

Some people take themselves so seriously that a single loss stops them forever.

If you play a game with a friend, what you will notice is that sometimes he or she clobbers you and sometimes you reign victorious.

You develop a strategy and sometimes it works out and sometimes it doesn't.

But if you play games, you keep playing and usually if you hang in there you may actually get a little better.

If you treated your life like a game, you would realize that the death phase is 100 percent certain for all of us so you might as well have fun in the meanwhile.

If you broke up with your boyfriend or girlfriend, never mind, there's always several million other people of the opposite sex who might be a better match. If your business fails, never mind, there's always another way to make a living. When it rains, never mind, sooner or later the sun will come out.

You can stop wasting your life force fretting over every little thing if you just wear it all a lot more lightly.

One of the best ways to approach the game of life more lightheartedly is to have fun competing with yourself.

Yesterday you walked three miles in so many minutes. Today you walk the same route just a little bit faster.

In this way, you build excitement about even the smallest challenges and avoid feeling so overwhelmed when things don't work out, when you actually lose or even when troubles pile up for seemingly long periods of time.

If you treated your entire life like a game, you would know the tough times never last and odds are sooner or later you will be back on top again.

Chapter 6

Give Yourself Permission to Create Your Best Possible Life

"Try and raise the vibration everywhere you go. Don't look for happiness, love, joy, beauty and peace. BE the happiness, love, joy, beauty and peace. Bring it to every space and situation you find yourself in. Make the world, room, day better because you are here." Amy Layne

Many of us have simply settled. We become half-way comfortable in life, and we stop striving for more.

This deadens our capacity and makes us give up, often before we have actually begun to live to our fullest capacity.

You can regain your chi by giving yourself permission to envision the best possible vision of your life.

Even if you feel you are already tremendously blessed, there is always more.

There could be even more happiness, even more love, even more joy, even more beauty and even more peace.

It doesn't mean your heart can't be full of true gratitude for what you already have, it just means that you can allow your soul to continue to grow.

Our soul actually wants to continue to grow.

Only our ego mind wants everything always comfortable and the same.

How do you give yourself permission to create your best possible life?

Ask yourself the following questions:

1. If your physical health could be even 2 percent better, what would you change? Two percent is a good place to look because it's such a small change that the amygdala, the fight, flight or freeze part of your brain, won't get too alarmed and shut you down.
2. If you could experience 2 percent more vitality in your life, what would you use it for?
3. If you could have 2 percent more happiness in your life, what would you like to enjoy?

If you feel ready, go for even bigger questions:

1. What is the one thing I can do in my life now that will most promote my spiritual growth?

2. If I could go anywhere, do anything and my success was totally assured, what would I do with myself?

If you can dream it, you can create it.

By allowing yourself to see all your possibilities, you will recognize that you are not stuck, that you still have choices.

Just recognizing your choices will put you back in a place of power, taking the steps to fulfill your soul purpose.

Chapter 7
Rewrite Your Story

"The past is not dead. In fact, it's not even past." William Faulkner

The story you tell yourself about literally any event in your past has an immediate effect on how you feel right now.

Think of biting into a lemon.

Did you notice how just thinking of biting into a lemon, you felt an immediate sour taste in your mouth? When we tell ourselves happy stories about what happened in our past, we produce our own feel-good neurotransmitters.

When we tell ourselves stories of trouble and woe, we can quite literally make ourselves feel exhausted and depressed in this moment even if the events we recall may have been long gone 20, 30, 40 and even 50 years ago.

Every time we retell our sorrowful story - whether we remember it that way in our own minds or tell it out loud to other people - we are quite literally creating the brain chemistry in this moment that makes us feel tired and depressed.

Nobody ever promised you that your life was going to be easy.

Just look at the Holmes and Rahe stress scale. The top 10 common stressors include: death of a spouse, divorce, marital separation, jail term, death of a close family member, personal injury, marriage, fired at work, marital reconciliation and retirement.

This list doesn't even include some of the rarer but unfortunate acts of fate - holocausts, tsunamis, world wars and famine.

It's amazing what we human beings can survive!

In asking you to rewrite your story, I am not asking you to change the facts.

What I am asking is that for your highest best interest to regain your energy that you look at it all from a totally different perspective.

Retell your story in such a way that you lose the feeling of a victim-perpetrator, reclaim your power and recognize that you actually chose, on a soul level, everything that has ever happened to you.

As you begin to see the blessings in each major life event, you will notice how your energy lifts.

When you rewrite your life story so that it's all good, so that you see only the blessings, you will no longer experience post traumatic stress disorder every time you think of your childhood or remember something unpleasant that actually happened.

Take your power back away from the so-called villains. Begin to restore your own unlimited energy and shift the way you feel inside.

Here's how you do this:

Step 1. Think of an unpleasant event. If this exercise feels overwhelming, start with something relatively mild or easy.

Step 2. As you recall your event, see if you can identify the main characters in your story. Who have you been calling the perpetrators, the villains or bad guys? Who have you been calling the victims?

Step 3. As you rethink your story, realize that everybody who took part in that event actually is a soul. Even if you don't quite understand what it was all for or all about, recognize that there may have been a higher spiritual purpose behind it.

Step 4. As you rethink your story, recall if you can any and all blessings that you personally received as a result of participating in or witnessing your story. Maybe you became wiser. Maybe you learned how to forgive. Maybe you let go of an old pattern, a person, place or thing that was no longer serving you. Maybe the trauma forced you to recognize your own power and choose to do something different with your life. Even if you can only think of just one thing, see if you can recognize how you are blessed as a result of what happened.

Step 5. Now as you recognize even one way that you were blessed by your story, start to see the larger picture. See how other people may have been blessed, how their lives were altered, how the whole picture was in fact one big blessing for everybody.

As you see the blessing, you begin to recognize that in terms of energy, we are all one. And it's all good and it's all God. There is nothing that has ever happened to you that ultimately was not for your highest good.

As you shift to this perception, notice how you feel more empowered. There's more life force available when we let go of our stories of victims and perpetrators.

Chapter 8
Take 100 Percent Responsibility

"You are the creator, enjoyer and destroyer of all you perceive." Sri Nisargatta Maharaj

Quite literally at a soul level, you have chosen everything that has ever happened to you.

It's as if your entire life has been set up as a spiritual self-study course, self-paced, so that you can learn whatever it is that you are here to learn.

I may need to learn one thing, you may need to learn something else.

When we take 100 percent responsibility for anything and everything that ever happens to us, we complete the cycle of playing the victim.

We take our power back.

Only when you take your power back and stop giving your power away to other people can you take 100 percent of your energy back.

If you have been blaming another person for anything that has happened, any feelings that you feel or literally any other aspect of your life, then you have given some of your chi away - even without recognizing it.

Giving your power away is a huge hidden cause of energy loss.

Here's how you can remedy the situation:

1. Make a list. On this list, write down the names of any people in your life you feel who have harmed you in any way.

2. Now take personal responsibility. Write down what you got out of every so-called harm. Often, we stay attached to the payoff of our anger, bitterness and resentment. We can come up with long, convincing stories about how it's actually all the other person's fault, that if that person just hadn't been so mean, our lives would be totally different. Recognize the juice you get out of giving your power away.

3. Now take your power back. In your mind, recognize what part you played in the drama. If you were observing the situation at the soul level, what actual blessings did you receive? Maybe you became stronger. Maybe you learned how to forgive. Maybe you are still learning how to forgive, but because of what

happened you have deeper insight. Literally visualize yourself taking your power and energy back from the person you had previously made responsible.

4. Now thank the soul of the people you once felt had wronged you. Use a simple forgiveness mantra:

I forgive (name the person)
(The person) forgives me.
I love (the person).
(The person) loves me.

Keep repeating the forgiveness mantra until the vibration between the two of you feels clear, open, calm and happy.

Recognize that you will not actually fully recover your vitality until you take 100 percent responsibility.

Chapter 9

Thoughts Are Actually Things

"Remember first, that everything you think, say and do is a reflection of what you have decided about yourself."
Neale Donald Walsh

Every time you think a thought, the neurons in your brain and all over your body begin to fire.

At the connection with other neurons there are chemical messengers called neurotransmitters that carry the energy and information of your thoughts.

When you think a thought or feel your emotions, you create these chemicals.

Therefore, thoughts are actually things.

When you habitually think positive thoughts, you boost your feel-good brain chemicals.

When you constantly drag yourself down with thoughts of worry, trouble, overwhelm and woe, you produce lots and lots and lots of stress hormones that deplete your feel-good brain chemicals.

When you say something unpleasant to another person, you literally change the energy between the two of you.

You can feel it.

Other people can experience it.

Many people are conscious enough that they would never say anything negative to other people, but they think negative thoughts about themselves all the time.

"I'm so fat," they think.

"This will never work out."

"Life is hard."

"Life is difficult."

Difficult, by the way, is the largest cult in the world!

When you recognize that thoughts are actually things, you can take 100 percent responsibility and catch yourself when you start to think negatively.

You may not always be able to come up with anything brilliantly inspiring, but you can probably do better than a negative thought.

If you recognize that you are constantly thinking negatively about yourself or others, you may benefit from re-examining your core beliefs.

You can start this way:

1. Write down your negative belief. For example, "My life sucks."
2. Then make a list of how you would like your life to be. Think of the opposite. What would it look? What would you hear other people saying to you if your life did not suck? What would you feel like?
3. Then come up with a simple statement of the positive. For example, "I LOVE my life."
4. Once you have your simple positive statement, whenever you hear your mind spouting out the same old negative thought, introduce the positive. "I LOVE my life." Even if you don't totally convince yourself initially by doing this, you will introduce a shadow of a doubt.

Continue this process until you have given up the habit of negative thinking and notice how your life essence has dramatically improved!

Chapter 10
Use Your Will Like a Sword

"Everything you do right now ripples outward and affects everyone. Your posture can shine your heart or transmit anxiety. Your breath can radiate love or muddy the room in depression. Your glance can awaken joy. Your words can inspire freedom. Your every act can open hearts and minds." David Deida

If you owned a sword, which you may or may not, depending on whether you practice fencing or tai chi, you would probably be very careful with it.

You probably wouldn't draw your sword at the slightest hint of attack.

You would keep your sword for special occasions when you really really need it.

One of the things that totally depletes your personal energy is trying to get everything done through the power of your will alone.

Will power is a fabulous thing. It is a gift when we are making an effort to lose weight, to complete a long, hard project, to take care of our babies in the middle of the night or to make the long drive home after a day at work.

As I have explained elsewhere in this book, every organ in your body has emotions associated with it.

And as you may recall, your adrenal glands - the ones that help you respond to stress - are associated with the emotion of will.

You can focus your willpower for the highest good of all, but if you are constantly pushing with your mind and using your will to try to control everything and everybody around you, you will soon find yourself feeling totally exhausted, even if you are eating organic food, juicing, meditating, exercising regularly, forgiving others and thinking positive thoughts.

Just as you would probably more than likely not use a sword in every situation, so should you learn not to use your will power to control every situation.

How do you do this differently?

The opposite of will power is not giving up, giving in or accepting failure.

The opposite of over using your will is going with the flow and allowing the universe, other people, events and information to unfold, trusting that everything happens in divine order.

If you allow yourself to discover life rather than pushing and shoving with your mind to make things happen the way you think they should, you will find yourself feeling much more free with your energy.

Use your will power just as you would a sword - carefully, thoughtfully and deliberately.

When we yield and flow with the frequencies all around us, we can end up preserving our own life force and feeling so much more free!

Chapter 11
Where Ever Your Attention Goes, Energy Flows

"Once you realize that all comes from within, that the world in which you live is not projected onto you, but by you, your fear comes to an end." Sri Nisargatta Maharaj

When you are working to build your personal chi, it is helpful to ask yourself where you place your attention.

Where ever your attention goes, energy flows.

If you are lying on the couch at home on a Saturday afternoon thinking about work, your chi is actually at the office.

If you are playing on the swing set with your children thinking about something that happened to your 20 years ago, that is where your chi actually is - in the past.

If you look around your house and see an object that reminds you of a childhood trauma, that is where your life force went - back to the place where you were deeply hurt.

When you truly wish to rebuild your vitality, you must watch where your mind goes.

When your mind goes back to the same times and places, over and over again, now you know where your life force has actually been draining into.

Choose to redirect your attention to all that uplifts you, all that inspires you, all that refreshes you and makes you laugh and brings you into the present moment.

If you catch yourself going into the past, call your spirit back.

If you catch yourself trying to rest and meandering into a lingering internal psychological turmoil, tell yourself it's not the time or place to resolve that right now.

Take a walk. Shift the frequency by redirecting your attention to something happening right now that feeds your soul. It could be your pet, a flower or just looking up at the sky!

You do not need to waste your vital essence on reliving the past or mulling over current traumas.

Yogis say that your mind is like a team of wild horses. Left undirected, your mind will meander everywhere.

Recognize that when you want to rebuild your animating force, you can place your attention with chi-giving people, places and activities.

Discover how you can easily restored simply by redirecting your mind.

Chapter 12
Your Fool Proof Thought

"Thoughts are energy - they are REAL and they have power." James Van Praagh

Because life isn't always easy, it's important to have a fool proof thought.

What do I mean by that?

Well, let's say you have to go to the dentist and they tell you that you have a cavity. Or you go to the doctor and they give you some diagnosis that you would rather not hear about.

Your first instinct may be go into some low frequency emotion, such as irritation, worry, anxiety or some other unfortunate tailspin.

The truth is that your personal frequency can only be as high as the quality of your thoughts and feelings.

When we allow ourselves to drop down into these low frequency energies, we feel very tired even if we haven't been digging ditches all day.

Therefore, it's always handy to have one single fool proof thought, a thought that every time you think it, you actually feel happy no matter what else is going on around you.

What would your fool proof thought be?

Pick something that has no negative charge on it whatsoever, no negative associations, only uplifting ones.

Chapter 13
Your Masks

"You have brains in your head. You have feet in your shoes. You can steer yourself in any direction you CHOOSE." Dr. Seuss

A mask is any role you play other than your true, authentic self.

You can also think of a mask as a defense system - a mode you go into whenever you don't feel totally safe to be yourself.

Your masks drag down your chi because they are not your highest or truest expression.

Think of a medieval soldier wearing armor to protect himself. How must that be, to walk around with so many layers of protection?

We also use masks to play roles based on what we believe we are expected to be.

Common masks include:

*Victim
*Saboteur
*Poor Me
*Interrogator
*Intimidator
*Aloof
*Misunderstood One
*Scapegoat
*Hero
*Clown
*Addict
*Enabler
*Damsel in Distress
*Homeless Person
*CEO
*Director
*Dictator
*Aristocrat
*King/ Queen
*Prince/ Princess
*Pauper
*Hopeless Case
*Visionary
*Poet

*Student
*Healer
*Rich Person
*Dilettante
*Expert
*Messiah
*Monk/ Nun
*Hermit
*Rebel
*Prostitute
*Thief
*Avenger
*Rescuer
*Priest/ Priestess
*Trickster
*Warrior

You may be able to think of many others.

At first glance, some of our masks may seem positive or even socially appropriate.

However, we deplete our chi whenever we are not being our true self.

Our true self may go through sorrow and woe, but our true self is never hopeless, lost, depressed or even broken.

We may feel all sorts of things, but the truth is that at our core soul level we are always unbroken and always at the perfect place on our life path, even if it appears on the outside to be an unmitigated disaster.

As you look over this list, ask yourself if there are common masks you tend to wear.

How do these roles hold back the true flow of your unlimited energy? You may put on certain masks with your child family - the one you grew up with.

You may put on other masks at work or with your friends.

You may even have an unhealthy relationship with yourself and tell yourself that there is something wrong with you, something missing in your life or that there is a gap that must be filled in order for you to feel complete.

The truth is that all these masks weigh down vibration because they impede the true flow of our life essence.

When you can drop all your masks - both with yourself and with others - you express your true self at all times.

It takes a lot less chi to be you than to be someone you are not, someone other people think you ought to be or someone you don't really want to be.

Be yourself at all times and see if you don't experience unlimited energy!

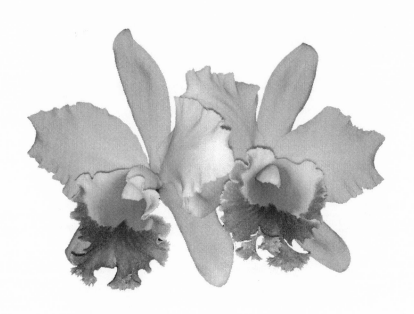

Book Five

Inspiring: Your Spiritual Body

Chapter 1

Connect To God Source

"Quantum physics thus reveals a basic oneness of the universe." Erwin Schrodinger

If you are totally honest with yourself, one day you will come to the realization that there is a limit to what you or anyone can know with your ego mind.

No matter how smart we are, how much we have practiced, how long we have studied or how many books we have read, there is an actual limit to what our intellect can perceive.

When we connect our total being to God, the unlimited source of all energy, however, we have the potential to connect to vibrations and information that can be of great service to ourselves as well as to others.

My recent book, *What Is Healing? Awaken Your Intuitive Power for Health and Happiness,* described how you can unlock your own intuitive abilities.

Although our own intelligence and personal prana may have a finite parameter, we can connect to God Source and enjoy a totally different experience of life.

When we connect to God through prayer, meditation and conscious intention to align our will to God's will, we allow the ever unfolding consciousness around us to be what it is and enjoy the play of light and love that surrounds us.

Even the Lord's Prayer acknowledges this recognition of humility and pronounces, "May thy will be done."

The Lord's Prayer:

Our Father, which art in heaven, Hallowed be thy Name. Thy Kingdom come. Thy will be done on earth, as it is in heaven. Give us this day our daily bread. And forgive us our trespasses, as we forgive them that trespass against us. And lead us not into temptation, But deliver us from evil. For thine is the kingdom,
The power, and the glory,
Forever and ever.
Amen.

When we connect to God Source, we can shift our perspective from seeing the world as "ain't it awful" to allowing the beautiful unfolding creation of life as it is meant to be.

When we shift into allowing, we can begin to feel gratitude for all that we have been blessed with.

Gratitude for God Source and for all our blessings is a huge reservoir of unlimited energy that is available to us at any time.

We can shift from the frequency of despair, hopelessness and giving up simply by recognizing the gift of our life itself.

When we look around at the people who surround us, the beauty of our planet, the sun, the moon and the stars, we recognize that the creation exceeds all bounds of expectation and is more wondrous than any single human mind could have personally imagined.

This sense of awe can be encompassed in the word, "Wow!"

Even if it's been years since you set foot in a church, a synagogue, mosque or meditation temple, you can honor the divine just by exclaiming "Wow" every time you recognize the immensity and enormity of all our blessings.

We can shift from focusing on what we don't have, all our pains and all the times we have truly suffered in our lives, to a recognition of how truly full of awe and wonder the experience has been.

"Wow!"

The truth is that it's all one energy. When we connect into it, through it and of it, we can connect to God Source easily and in so doing joyfully experience unlimited energy.

Chapter 2

Cord Connections

"Physics is like sex: sure, it may give some practical results, but that's not why we do it." Richard Feynman

One of the issues that affects our vitality, often without our conscious awareness, is the cord connections we have with other people.

In your body, you have energy vortexes called chakras.

When we have close intimate connections with other people, such as with our children, mothers and fathers as well as people with whom we have had sex, we form invisible cords that connect us through our chakras.

An intuitive healer can easily read the quality of any relationship by reading the cords between two people.

When we truly love others, we connect cords from heart to heart.

In addition to the cords from heart to heart, we also connect at the other chakras as well.

When we connect at the first chakra, we derive a sense of family and identity.

When we connect at the second chakra, we feel a sexual attraction.

When we connect at the third chakra, we are empathetic with the other person's feelings.

When we connect at the heart chakra, we truly love the other person.

When we connect at the fifth chakra, we have a lot to talk about and can speak our truth.

When we connect at the sixth chakra, we share our vision of the world.

When we connect at the seventh chakra, we experience a strong spiritual connection.

When we connect deeply with another person on all the levels, we have a very deep and rich, mutually rewarding relationship.

There can be many cords going back and forth between two people.

Sometimes you may connect with another person one way but not in others.

For example, you may enjoy great conversation but not feel sexually attracted. You may feel a soul connection with someone you have never met, even if you have a totally different vision of life.

These cord connections literally feed our energy.

Haven't you felt tremendously energized by a great evening of friendship and conversation?

Some people you just need to hang out with and all of a sudden you feel tremendously more at peace.

Here are a few suggestions about how you can manage the cords between yourself and other people:

1. When you are complete with another person, such as when you break off a relationship, it's important that you cut the cords. People who have been divorced even 12 years before may still be energetically connected to their ex-spouse, keeping their energy in the past and unable to move forwards.
2. From a psychic perspective, these cords look like translucent garden hoses. They convey energy and information between two people on an unspoken basis. It's part of why you can know what other people know, feel what they feel, hear what they hear and see what they see.
3. To cut the cords, visualize the other person in front of you. In your mind or out loud, speak your truth. Say whatever it is that you need to say to his or her soul in order to be complete. Then visualize yourself

unplugging your cords out of his or her chakras. Cut the cords from him or her into your chakras.

4. If you are away from your loved one, you can send rainbows from your chakras to his or her chakras. This is a lovely way to continue to feel connected. This will support both of you during your absence.

5. If a person has actually died, it is very important that you allow him or her to move on. If you fail to allow the other person to move on, this may continue to drag your vibration to a great degree. Cut the cords with all your loved ones who have passed on.

Chapter 3

Forgiveness Frees Your Prana

"The scarcest resource is not oil, metals, clean air, capital, labor, or technology. It is our willingness to listen to each other and learn from each other and to seek the truth rather than seek to be right." Donella Meadows

Many spiritual people know that it's a good idea to forgive others but they really have no clue how to go about that.

When we hold onto resentment, bitterness and grudges, those energies literally lodge somewhere in your body.

Lack of forgiveness may hurt your heart, it may harden your arteries, and it may clog your liver and gallbladder. It may shut down your breath and deplete your brain chemistry.

You can begin to forgive others first by recognizing that forgiveness frees YOU.

It doesn't change what happened.

What it does is change the frequency you are currently experiencing as a result of the story you have told yourself about what you thought happened in the past.

If you don't forgive, your story lives on and on in your cells, making you feel sick and literally exhausted.

When we are willing to forgive, we are willing to give up our nasty habit of bitterness, resentment and grudges.

We are willing to let go of the story that somehow, some way, we were actually a victim and not a full, 100 percent participating and responsible actor in our own drama.

When we let go of that story, we recognize that other people are not actually villains.

They are humans also - just like us, they are not perfect.

They are practicing being human, and even if they don't have the whole thing down pat just yet, when we are totally honest, neither do we, really.

A great way to begin is with a simple mantra.

When we become angry and stressed, we act sort of stupid and can lose our higher judgment, so having simple techniques to turn to when we are not at our best is generally quite helpful.

I forgive (name the person).
(The person) forgives me.
I love (the person).
(The person) loves me.

In the Bible, Matthew 18:21-22, Jesus was once asked how many times we should forgive someone:

"Then Peter came to Jesus and asked, 'Lord, how many times shall I forgive my brother or sister who sins against me? Up to seven times?'

"Jesus answered, 'I tell you, not seven times, but seventy-seven times.'"

Even though we are directed to forgive again and again, we sometimes wonder if there ought to be a limit to how many times we should forgive someone.

Repeat the mantra - either out loud or silently - until the energy surrounding the situation feels totally shifted.

Whether it takes you seventy repetitions or many days, weeks or months of repetitions doesn't actually matter.

Each time you affirm your willingness to forgive, you are reclaiming layers and layers of your own life force.

You are raising your own vibration to one of acceptance of all that is.

In so doing, you will experience unlimited energy.

Chapter 4
Joy

"Quantum physics tells us that nothing that is observed is unaffected by the observer. That statement, from science, holds enormous and powerful insight. It means that everyone sees a different truth, because everyone is creating what they see." Neale Donald Walsh

Of all the kinds of energies that we can experience as human beings, joy is the highest vibration.

The more joy you can give yourself permission to experience in your life, the more you will be blessed with unlimited energy.

Many people waste their lives getting and spending, working, toiling, worrying, pushing and shoving without stopping to pause and really feel moments of true joy.

Where can you find joy?

In a leaf falling from the sky.
In a feather you discover lying unpretentiously in the street.
In the smile of a stranger.
In a hot bath.
In a cup of tea.

Another word for joy is ecstasy - sublime moments that seem to transcend time and space.

You experience joy by being in the moment with whatever is present.

Yes, you can go on a fancy vacation, travel the world and admire its wonders, but you can also take the time to feel joyful where ever you are in your everyday life, no ticket required.

Create the space in your life to experience whatever is happening with no rushing, no editorial commentary with your mind.

Just be with yourself and discover what happens.

You can give yourself permission to discover joy in unexpected places.

It's here, ever present, if you just pause to experience it!

Chapter 5
Listen To Your Angels

"It is important to realize that in physics today, we have no knowledge what energy is. We do not have a picture that energy comes in little blobs of a definite amount." Richard Feynman

Everybody has angels, whether you call them that or not.

Some people prefer to call them your spiritual guides.

Whether you call them your angels or call them your spiritual guides, what they really are is your team of high frequency beings here to guide, protect and direct you in every aspect of your life.

Often we waste a lot of our personal life force making disastrous although well-intentioned and even highly informed decisions.

We may do a lot of research, consult a lot of experts and still come up with a very stupid choice.

On the other hand, if there is some really important decision to make, we can save ourselves a lot of energy by simply consulting our divine management team, our spiritual board of directors, who actually have our highest best interests at heart with no ulterior motives.

A great time to have an uninterrupted conversation with your angels is in the middle of the night.

Although we can talk to our angels at any time of night or day, we often get busy and discover that it's easier to listen in the dead of the night when there is nothing else to do, no other interference.

Listening to your own guidance saves you so much energy because you will invariably be directed to the people, places, and situations that are for your highest good.

This saves a huge amount of time and possibly even money and effort.

How do you listen to your angels?

1. Set aside quiet time to be by yourself.
2. Pull out your journal of simply a piece of paper.
3. Say a prayer and call in your angels. You could simply say:

Angel spirit guides, I am ready to listen. I am asking for your guidance at this time.

4. At the top of your piece of paper, write: "*My angels say.*" Then begin writing as if you are simply taking dictation. Get your ego mind out of the way and simply write down what you hear. Don't judge it - just write it. After awhile, your dictation will come to an end.

5. Once you are completely finished taking dictation, then go back and read what your angels had to say. You probably heard it the first time, but now you can go back to reflect.

Over time, as you consult your divine management team, you will see for yourself what their track record is.

As you come to trust the information you receive through listening, you may find that your angels never steer you wrong.

Chapter 6

Meditation, A Way to Empty That Which Is Too Full

"Empty your mind. Be formless, shapeless like water. You put water into a cup, it becomes the cup. Put it in a teapot, water can flow or creep or drip or crash. Be water my friend." Bruce Lee

Although meditation is now scientifically proven to have numerous health benefits, one of the greatest blessings of this practice is that it is a wonderful way to empty that which is too full.

When you take the time to empty your mind, your guidance can slip through.

You set down the weight of all your thoughts.

You restore yourself by simply being.

When we are too yang - too active, too hot, too full - we can restore balance to our energy system by being yin.

Yin energy is quiet and still.

Meditation is the epitome of a yin practice.

Whether you sit or lie down is irrelevant - either way you connect with the slower earth frequencies in order to make yourself a conduit to receive divine flow.

The irony is that to experience unlimited energy all you have to do is empty yourself completely of all your stress, worry, and thought and rediscover the strength of your own center.

Chapter 7
Negative Spiritual Energy

"The reality we can put into words is never reality itself."
Werner Heisenberg

It's all one energy.

Within that one energy, however, are different vibrations. High frequency vibrations uplift us. Low frequencies make us sick and depressed.

You can use muscle testing to determine the frequency of any energy - whether that vibration is a person, a flower essence, a food, a drug, a supplement or any living being.

For convenience sake, we humans tend to put labels on things - if your dinner companion asks for pepper, you probably know not to give him salt.

One of the kinds of frequencies that tend to drag us down is negative spiritual energies. There are several different kinds of negative spiritual energies:

*Witchcraft spells
*Voodoo
*Black magic
*Satanic entities
*Emotional turmoil entities
*Earthbound entities
*Gloom, doom, and disaster
*Negative spirit attachments
*Fear entities
*Curses

It's all here. The angelic is here, the demonic is here.

You are like one of those old time radio sets - the ones where you could roll the dial.

You can tune into public radio, rap, easy listening, rock n' roll, classical, heavy metal, New Age, jazz or country music - you name it.

The angelic and the demonic are here, and you get to choose what you set your frequency to.

Often people who have negative spiritual attachments are very good, kind-hearted people. They could have become attached from having a literal hole in their energy field.

If you have been suffering from any mental illness, lifelong physical illness or severe, unrelenting pain it is a good idea to check for low frequency energies.

You have an energy grid that surrounds you.

When we are healthy, this energy grid is complete, but sometimes, just like old socks, the energy grid may become thin or develop holes.

You may be a very good person, but if you leave your door open at night then everybody and their brother can come in.

If you feel you may have a negative spiritual attachment, seek professional help. I do not recommend that you try to remove it yourself.

Chapter 8
Parallel Universe Integration

"Stress is caused by being here but wanting to be there."
Eckhart Tolle

A somewhat unusual but possible cause of chronic fatigue is parallel universe integration.

You are a soul. You have a body.

Your soul has been around a long time - much longer than just in this life time with the experience of just this particular human body.

Sometimes what happens is that your soul gets confused and is trying to experience two lifetimes at the same time.

Whatever is going on in the other lifetime may drag you down in this lifetime - even if nothing is actually wrong in this lifetime.

For example, you could be literally starving in another life but in this life you could have plenty of food all around you but you are always hungry and there is no rational medical explanation for it.

To restore your unlimited energy, you want your soul to bring 100 percent of you into this lifetime, into this now, so that you can live just one lifetime at a time.

Set your intention to pull yourself into present reality and notice how your energy improves.

Chapter 9
Soul Agreements

"The soul doesn't absorb negativity by accident, always by choice." Rachel Wolchin

Often as human beings we misunderstand the nature of our relationships with other people.

Someone may hurt you so deeply in so many ways that you spend the rest of your life in different forms of therapy trying to get over what happened.

In such cases, where you have been hurt very deeply and so much of your life force is devoted to reliving, analyzing and controlling your reactions to the previous situation, it is very helpful to understand the nature of soul agreements.

A soul agreement is an agreement that you made with another soul before you were born.

Sometimes these soul agreements are mutual.

I am going to help you with something and you are going to help me also.

Sometimes soul agreements are one way.

I am going to help you, but it's O.K. that I don't appear to get anything out of it.

You are going to help me, and it's also O.K. that you don't appear to get anything out of it.

If we look at it from the soul perspective, it's all sacred.

We can tie up so much vital force trying to make all the relationships in our lives feel like 50-50, as if we were all back in grade school.

We waste chi expecting life to be fair when we can see things instead from a broader perspective and recognize the soul agreements that we have made.

Here's how you can recognize soul agreements:

1. If there is someone in your life who you haven't been able to understand completely, visualize your soul and their soul having a conversation.
2. As you visualize the soul of the other person, ask the other person's soul to explain to you whether or not you have a soul agreement.
3. If you do have a soul agreement, ask if it is mutual or one way.

4. Once you discover what kind of soul agreement you have, ask what the purpose of the soul agreement is.

5. If you would like to be complete with the agreement and move on, ask the soul of the other person what you need to do, say, be or have in order to be complete.

6. Finally, thank the soul of the other person for whatever role it is that they have played in your life. Bless the other person and feel blessed by them.

Chapter 10

The Parts You Left Behind

"An eye for an eye only ends up making the whole world blind." Mahatma Gandhi

Often in life we experience a trauma. This trauma could be physical, such as a car wreck. It could be energetic, such as the separation from a loved one. It could be emotional, such as the loss of a pet. It could be mental, such as a blow to our ego. It could be spiritual, such as a wound so deep that it goes to the depths of our soul.

At theses points in time, we lose aspects of our true self.

You may be feeling low in vitality because you have lost a significant, meaningful part of yourself.

It's as if energetically a fragment breaks off and flies somewhere in space, like a chip off an old China plate.

It's available somewhere out in the universe but not actually attached to us.

To restore our unlimited energy now, we need to retrieve the part of us that have been left behind. Some people call this process a soul retrieval.

If you are feeling low in life essence, ask yourself the following questions?

1. Have I experienced a trauma in my life that caused me to lose an important aspect of my personality?
2. Have I gone through a period where I gradually lost my sense of meaning and joy?
3. Are there activities that I always felt I was meant to do that are no longer part of my life? Many people grew up longing to be a musician, or a writer, or an explorer. As they grew into adulthood, they gave up what they considered to be silly dreams but in doing so they also lost their sense of joy and wonder.

You can do a healing on yourself to return, refresh and restore all your soul fragments. In so doing, you restore your full energy.

Step 1. Sit or lie down in a comfortable position in a place where you feel safe and relaxed.

Step 2. Call on all your angels and spiritual guides. These are spiritual beings who have been with you throughout this lifetime and possibly beyond that. Even if you have never communicated with them before, they are there and they are your team, always looking out for you. They already know best how to heal you.

Step 3. Say a prayer:

Dear God, I call on all my angels and all my spiritual guides. I ask that all fragments of my soul that have been lost be now returned, restored and reintegrated in a healthy, easy way.

I ask that this be done for the highest good of all. Thank you God, thank you God. Amen.

Step 4. Perhaps you know the part or parts of you that were lost. It could be your happy self, your musician self, your artist or your brave explorer. As you say your prayer, visualize a picture of how you will be now that you are whole and complete.

What actions will you take when all of you is restored to a feeling of wholeness?

What would you need to do, be or have in order to reintegrate the parts you left behind?

If you lost your musician, maybe you might take up music again. If you lost your artist, maybe you would return to painting. If you lost your explorer, you might plan a trip, even if it's out West touring with your dog in an old truck.

Take the steps necessary to be present with your whole self now and enjoy the fullness of your life.

Chapter 11
Your Life Is the Meaning

"Your vibe speaks volumes louder than any words could ever speak." Dulce Ruby Peralta

One of the ways to be truly happy in life, which will bless you with unlimited energy, is to discover the meaning of your life.

Mahatma Gandhi was once asked what the meaning of his life was. "My life is my message," he said.

Often we expect that the meaning our life has to be somehow bigger than us, like finding the cure for cancer.

Maybe the meaning of your life is sitting under a tree, enjoying the sunshine, petting your dog, making a meal for your family, giving and receiving hugs, loving the people you call friends and family.

As we connect with our spiritual self, we can recognize just how profound each of these small, significant acts may be.

When we sit under a tree, doing apparently nothing, we bring our frequency into the present moment.

When we are in the present moment, our prana is not dredging through our past or fearfully anticipating the future.

We experience more chi in the now than in any other time in space.

When we pet our dog, we harmonize our EKG and our EEG with the frequency of love, which is the most powerful healing force in the universe. Even if we aren't thinking about love, we are in the feeling of it and living and experiencing and sharing that specific vibration, which lifts up not only ourselves but everyone around us.

When we make a meal for our family, we put our own chi into blessing all that nurtures our loved ones. We set a silent unspoken intention that everyone around us be fulfilled by our small act of kindness.

When we take the time to enjoy our friends and family, we lift up everyone around us, as easily as if we were tossing a small child into the air.

The social connectedness acts like a glue that mends not just a few moments but can last a lifetime in remembered words and deeds of thoughtfulness.

Your life need not have a huge meaning in order to be replete with meaning.

As you grab on to the chi present and available in all these sweet moments, you can enjoy the ecstasy of unlimited energy.

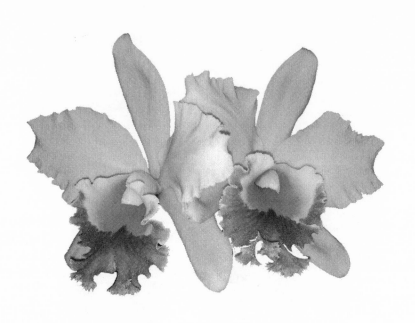

Conclusion

Chapter 1
You, The Ultimate Energy Manager

"Life is all about perception. Positive versus negative. Whichever you choose will affect and more than likely reflect your outcomes." Sonya Teclai

If you have ever worked for a large corporation, what you may notice is that many people have very fancy job titles.

Me, I am a medical intuitive healer, but I also do everything.

I am the Chief Sanitation Officer, as I take out the trash from office.

I am the Orchid Care Specialist, as I carefully water and tend to the orchids in the studio where I do my healing work.

I am the Dog Walker, Chief Dog Psychologist and Dog Bathing Expert, as I give my dog Belle her bath every week, since she comes to work with me and I would prefer for her to be clean when she greets my clients.

In addition to all your job titles, whether you realize it or not, you are your own Ultimate Energy Manager.

You get to decide whether or not you are going to live, breathe and work at a very high vibration.

You decide whether you put dead, low vibration food in your mouth or not.

You get to choose whether or not you practice energy exercise, breath work, whether or not you hang on to your negative emotions and old faulty beliefs. You choose whether or not you hold on to your bitterness, anger and resentment or whether you let go and forgive everyone for everything.

You choose whether or not you can allow the world to be whatever it will be or whether you will try to push and shove with your mind, trying to control every little aspect with your own personal vitality.

Once you recognize that you are actually in charge of all this, you have the power within you to make yourself feel 100 percent better.

My prayer is that this book has brought you insight into ways you can experience ultimate energy.

Chapter 2
Blessings from Heaven

"Happiness is your nature. It is not wrong to desire it. What is wrong is seeking it outside when it is inside." Ramana Maharshi

Taking just a few ideas from this book can bless you with ultimate unlimited energy.

Once you experience unlimited energy, you will do whatever it takes to preserve it.

You will eat well.

You will rest well.

You will exercise in very intelligent ways that actually make you feel better.

You will deal with your emotions as they arise, and think the best possible thought in every situation.

You will listen to your angels for guidance and become more efficient by following divine direction.

I would love to hear your stories about how this book has blessed you with unlimited energy.

If you are just reading this book for the first time and want to hear how other people have rebuilt their life energy, feel free to read testimonials from my clients at the following links:
http://catherinecarrigan.com/testimonials/
http://unlimitedenergynow.com/testimonials/

Please email me at catherine@catherinecarrigan.com to let me know how you have been blessed with more vitality, and let me know all the life goals that you have been able to accomplish as a result.

I want to hear how your life has been blessed and how you have become a blessing to everyone around you as a result of your unlimited energy.

Blessings from heaven! Let's all share in the abundance that is available to all of us.

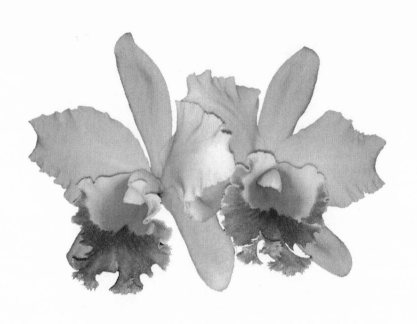

Appendix

Chapter 1

How to Ask For Guidance

"Energy is contagious, positive and negative alike. I will forever be mindful of what and who I am allowing into my space." Alex Elle

You can save yourself a tremendous amount of mental wear and tear by asking for guidance.

No matter how smart you are, how well educated you are, how many years of experience you may have in your business, there is a limit to what your ego mind is capable of knowing.

No matter how great you are at researching, there is a limit to what your intellect can figure out.

Before you begin, you must be in neutral.

When you are in neutral, you are open to receiving whatever information comes through. You are not *fine -*

fucked up, insecure, neurotic, or emotional. You are calm and at peace.

Here's a few great ways to get to neutral:

1. Spend time in meditation. Meditation clears your mind and allows the space for your guidance to come through. I often receive my best information after meditating.
2. Make sure you are properly hydrated. Simply being dehydrated will increase the tension in your central nervous system. Drink water.
3. Practice yoga, tai chi or qi gong to clear your acupuncture meridians, chakras and breath channels.
4. Cross crawl. Bring your opposite hand to your opposite knee. Cross crawling integrates the right and left hemispheres of your brain, which allows you to see things from a whole-brain perspective.
5. Breathe. If you are holding your breath, you are in some degree of fight or flight.
6. Relax your jaw. If your jaw is clenched, you are locked in your ego mind.
7. Say a prayer from your heart asking for information for the highest good of all. Here's a good example:

Heavenly Father,
Angels, spiritual guides,
I call on you at this time and ask you to guide me.
Please open my mind and direct me.

Give me the information that I need at this time to make choices for the highest good of all.
Thank you God, thank you angels, thank you spiritual guides. Amen.

Once you are in neutral, any one of the following techniques will work.

Whether you are muscle testing yourself, using a pendulum, using your body as a pendulum or getting another person to muscle test you, the truth is that you are asking universal source. The technique does not actually matter. Just find what works for you!

Chapter 2
Self Testing Techniques

"Energy rightly applied and directed can accomplish anything." Nellie Bly

1. Two-finger loop. With your left hand, bring your thumb and pointer finger together. With your right hand, bring your thumb and pointer finger together inside the loop you just made with your left hand. Think of a question with a yes or no answer. Then pull your right hand loop. If your answer is YES, the loop will stay closed. If your answer is NO, your right fingers will slide through the loop.

2. Single hand finger cross. If you are right-handed, use your right hand. Think of a yes or no question. Take the middle finger and cross it over your pointer finger. If your answer is YES, your fingers will stay stuck

together. If your answer is NO, your middle finger will slide across the pointer finger.

3. Use your head. Imagine that your head is a floating ball on the tip of your neck. Think of a yes or no question. If your answer is YES, your head will tilt slightly forward. If your answer is NO, your head will tilt backwards.

4. Two finger rub. If you are right handed, use your right hand. Think of a question. Then rub the pad of your middle finger on top of the pad of your thumb. If you receive a YES answer, your fingers will seem to stick together. If you receive a NO answer, your fingers will seem to slide apart.

5. Thymus test. This works if you are doing a general test to see if a food, supplement or other substance is beneficial for your overall well-being. Stand up. Hold the substance at your thymus, the center of your chest. If it is something that will strengthen you, your body will move towards it. If it is something that will weaken you, your body will naturally move away from it.

6. Snap. Think of a yes or no question. Snap your fingers. If you receive a YES, you will hear a crisp sound. If you receive a NO, the sound will be dull or silent.

Chapter 3
Using a Pendulum

"Every single one of us is a unique vibration in a beautiful symphony of infinite creation." Gordana Biernat

You can purchase a pendulum very inexpensively.

You can certainly find pendulums made from beautiful crystals, but these may need the energy cleared because most crystals hold vibrations.

If you are purchasing a pendulum for the first time, I recommend you buy a metal one.

Or you could simply tie a string on to the circle of an eye bolt screw.

In a pinch, you can use the decorative end of a necklace.

Frankly, the device doesn't matter.

Step 1. Get clear on a yes and a no. Start by swinging your pendulum back and forth in a vertical direction.

Step 2. Say out loud, "Show me a YES." Usually the pendulum will swing in a clockwise direction with a YES.

Step 3. Say out loud, "Show me a NO." Usually the pendulum will swing counter clockwise with a NO.

Step 4. Once you are clear on the signals for yes and no, you can begin to ask questions.

A pendulum can also be used to show the quality of chi in any object.

For example, if you hold a pendulum over a plate of junk food, microwaved food or fast food, you will notice that the pendulum probably stays either still, meaning that there is no life force in it and will not bring you more life force, or actually move counter clockwise, which means that so-called food is toxic for your body.

On the other hand, if you place a pendulum over a plate of homemade, organic food that has been prayed over, you will see the pendulum swing clockwise in a large circle, meaning the food is tremendously nourishing and will actually increase your life force.

Chapter 4
Using Your Body as a Pendulum

"Our entire biological system, the brain and the earth itself, work on the same frequencies." Nikola Tesla

You can also use your whole body as a pendulum.

Step 1. Stand up comfortably in the middle of a room.

Step 2. Say out loud, "Show me a YES." More than likely, you will rock forward slightly.

Step 3. Say out loud, "Show me a NO." When you receive a no, you will feel your weight shifting backwards.

Step 4. Once you have calibrated YES and NO, you can begin to ask questions.

It is a good idea to start asking for guidance with yes and no questions.

As you progress, you may notice that you are hearing, seeing, feeling or simply just knowing the answers as you go along.

When this happens, you have opened up your psychic gifts and can begin receiving even higher quality information.

If you would like to open your psychic gifts, you may want to read my recent Amazon No. 1 bestselling book, *What Is Healing? Awaken Your Intuitive Power for Health and Happiness* (Atlanta: Total Fitness, 2013).

Chapter 5
Muscle Testing with Another Person

"Concerning matter, we have been all wrong. What we have called matter is energy, whose vibration has been so lowered as to be perceptible to the senses. There is no matter." Albert Einstein

Step 1. Both parties must be in neutral. Clear your personal chi before you begin.

Step 2. The person being tested stands or sits in a comfortable position. This person is the Subject. The person who is doing the muscle testing stands or sits next to them. This person is the Tester.

Step 3. The Tester must have two points of contact with the Subject or chi may be drained from one or both people during the muscle testing process. This is because prana always flows from highest to lowest potential. The Subject extends one arm to the side. The Tester places one hand on the opposite should and two fingers two inches above the wrist of the extended arm.

Step 4. Calibrate a yes and a no. Have the Subject say "YES." The Tester presses down gently, using two ounces of pressure two inches above the wrist. The Subject's arm should drop. Have the subject say "NO." The Subject's arm should hold strong. I usually also like to add several other steps to the calibration process. I have the Subject say, "I AM (their name)," which should hold strong, and then say another "I am (another name," which should test weak. I also like to have the person shut their eyes, saying "NO" and "YES." If any of this leads to confused responses, both parties need to clear their energies once again.

Step 5. Ask YES or NO questions. I like to add in "highest best interests." For example, "It is in my highest best interests to eat a hot fudge sundae today" will probably evoke a different response than "Can I eat a hot fudge sundae?"

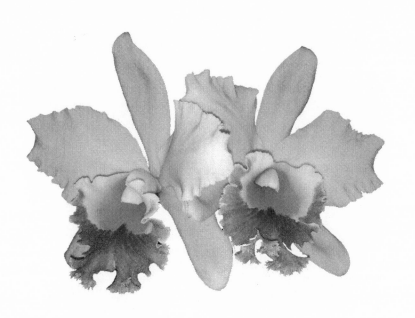

About The Author
Catherine Carrigan

I have the ability to get to the heart of the matter and figure out what will actually work to make you radiantly healthy.

Hi, my name is Catherine Carrigan.

I am a medical intuitive healer.

The average person who comes to see me has seen at least seven other practitioners – medical doctors, psychologists, psychiatrists, chiropractors, shamans, homeopaths, physiotherapists, nutritionists, herbalists, acupuncturists – you name it.

I offer a comprehensive system that begins with figuring out what is actually going on with you and then putting together a personalized plan that empowers you to achieve levels of health that you may not have even thought possible.

I do not need to see you or put my hands on you to know what is wrong or what will make you better.

I have a passion for healing, and I can teach you how to become healthy using natural methods, including the very best of therapeutic exercise, nutrition and energy medicine.

You can connect with me on Facebook at https://www.facebook.com/catherinecarriganauthor

Follow me on Twitter at https://twitter.com/CSCarrigan

Read my blog at www.catherinecarrigan.com

Follow my website at www.unlimitedenergynow.com

Connect with me on LinkedIn at:
www.linkedin.com/in/catherinecarrigan/

Sign up for my newsletter at:
http://visitor.r20.constantcontact.com/manage/optin?v=0 01PTUI55zVN-iNOxZk5SNQKwTDWN_rJO255xm7nU j20MlJleYyNmpCQzG4L5gy5tcrk9Ujk2zW9GFT3LEo1y c2fkG3uErNj0GSr7zNs5jqBFU%3D

You can read testimonials from my clients here:
http://catherinecarrigan.com/testimonials/
http://unlimitedenergynow.com/testimonials/

Training in Fitness

- Certified Personal Fitness Trainer: A.C.E. certified in Personal Fitness Training.

- Corrective High-Performance Exercise Kinesiologist Practitioner (C.H.E.K. Practitioner), Level I: Chek Institute.
- Certified Group Exercise Instructor: A.C.E. certified in Group Exercise.
- A.C.E. Specialty Recognitions: Strength training and Mind-Body Fitness.
- Exercise Coach, Chek Institute.
- Certified Yoga Teacher: 500-hour Yoga Teacher through Lighten Up Yoga. Six 200-hour certifications through Integrative Yoga Therapy, the White Lotus Foundation, and the Atlanta Yoga Fellowship, Lighten Up Yoga and Erich Schiffmann teacher training, twice.
- Practitioner of Qi Gong, Chinese martial arts.
- Certified Older Adult Fitness Trainer through the American Institute of Fitness Educators.

Training in Nutrition

- Food Healing Level II Facilitator.
- Holistic Lifestyle Coach, though the Chek Institute, Level 3.
- Certified Sports Nutritionist through the American Aerobics Association International/International Sports Medicine Association.
- Author, *Healing Depression: A Holistic Guide* (New York: Marlowe and Co., 1999), a book discussing

nutrition and lifestyle to heal depression without drugs.
- Schwarzbein Practitioner though Dr. Diana Schwarzbein, M.D., expert in balancing hormones naturally.

Training in Healing

- Specialized Kinesiology, through Sue Maes of London, Ontario, Canada.
- Self Empowerment Technology Practitioner.
- Brain Gym, Vision Circles and Brain Organization instructor through the Educational Kinesiology Foundation.
- Certified Touch for Health practitioner.
- Thai Yoga Body Therapy.
- Flower Essence Practitioner.
- Reiki Master, Usui tradition.
- Life Coaching through Sue Maes' Mastering Your Knowledge Mentorship Program and Peak Potentials.
- Medical Intuitive Readings and Quantum Healing.

Other Training

- Health and fitness columnist.
- Playwright of 12 plays, 3 produced in New York City.
- Past Spokesperson, the Depression Wellness Network.
- Phi Beta Kappa graduate of Brown University.
- Former national spokesperson for Johnson & Johnson.
- Owner and co-host, Total Fitness Radio Show.

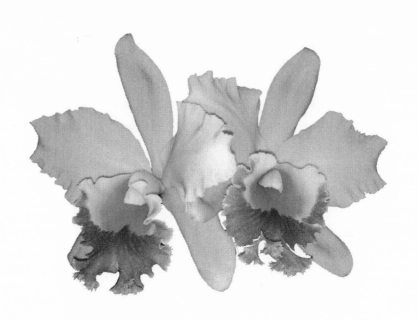

About The Cover Artist
Mynzah Osiris

Mynzah Osiris is a spiritual artist who experienced a kundalini awakening in November of 2008.

In this lifetime, he has had experiences in the U.S. Marine Corps and a local sheriff's department.

You can view his lovely artwork at www.mynzah.com and follow his imagery at http://www.pinterest.com/mynzah/.

Mynzah creates digital art that is inspired by love and remembrance. The colors of his art usually are vivid so he can see them because he is color deficient. Sacred Geometry, Ancient History and Evolution of Consciousness are important factors into his creations as well.

In addition to the joy of creating digital art, he also writes poetry, creates jewelry and plays drums and Native American flute. He enjoys expressing himself in an authentic, artistic and positive way.

The art Mynzah creates is set with an intention that is adhered to a collective unified vision. He envisions a world awake to the internal truth of Oneness. Through the various artistic expressions by Mynzah, his intention is to help facilitate the expansion of consciousness from separation and fear, to remembrance, unification and love.

Made in the USA
Charleston, SC
18 December 2014